The Narcissistic and Borderline Disorders

An Integrated Developmental Approach

By

James F. Masterson, M.D.

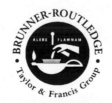

Brunner-Routledge
New York & London

Published by
Brunner-Routledge
29 West 35th Street
New York, NY 10001

Published in Great Britain
Brunner-Routledge
11 New Fetter Lane
London EC4P 4EE

Brunner-Routledge is an imprint of the Taylor & Francis Group

Library of Congress Cataloging in Publication Data

Masterson, James F.
  The narcissistic and borderline disorders.

  Bibliography: p.
  Includes index.
    1. Narcissism.   2. Pseudoneurotic schizophrenia.   3. Personality,
Disorders of.
I. Title.   [DNLM: 1. Narcissism.   2. Personality disorders
3. Borderline personality disorders.
WM 460.5.E3 M423n]
RC553.N36M37   616.85'82   81-38540
ISBN 0-87630-292-4   AACR2

MANUFACTURED IN THE UNITED STATES OF AMERICA

17 18 19 20 MV MV 0 9 8 7

Contents

Introduction

A borderline patient reported: "I have such a poor self-image and so little confidence in myself that I can't decide what I want, and when I do decide, I have even more difficulty doing it."

A narcissistic patient reported: "I was denied promotion to chief executive by my board of directors, although my work was good, because they felt I had poor relations with my employees. When I complained to my wife, she agreed with the board, saying my relations with her and the children were equally bad. I don't understand. I know I'm more competent than all these people."

These two statements vividly illustrate the wide spectrum of the psychopathology of the self (narcissism), which ranges from the deficient emotional investment in the self seen in the borderline to the pathologic overinvestment of the self seen in the narcissistic patient. Many a borderline patient reports being green with envy at the façade of self-confidence exhibited by the narcissistic patient.

Ignoring these key differences and seeing both disorders as one has created endless confusion (58-63). This book describes the differences between the two disorders in developmental level, intrapsychic structure and clinical picture and details the differences in therapeutic technique required to treat them.

The quantum leap in the understanding of the psychopathology of borderline and narcissistic disorders which has occurred in recent years has improved therapeutic techniques and led to better clinical results. This new understanding has sprung from, as well as stimulated, excursions into theory regarding how early development affects character formation: What factors are essential to normal development? What goes wrong with this course of events to produce a borderline syndrome or a narcissistic personality disorder?

The hypotheses for these theories have derived from three sources: (a) the psychoanalytic treatment of children; (b) anamnestic reconstructions from the analysis of borderline and narcissistic adults; and (c) direct child-observation research by analytic observers of normal children—in vivo, so to speak—as they passed through these early phases of development. Any theory of the borderline and narcissistic disorders, to have maximum explanatory power and appropriate and close clinical "fit," should utilize both reconstruction from analysis and child observation studies of normal development. Even though these two sources differ in the nature of the data obtained and the method of study, their findings reinforce each other. Any theory, therefore, should comprise concepts derived from the developmental theory of symbiosis and separation-individuation (1, 2, 74, 76), as observed and described in normal development, as well as the pathology of the separation-individuation (72, 83, 96) process which produces various developmental arrests.

Most psychoanalytic authors (43-50; 58-63) emphasize only one source, the analytic evidence, to the exclusion of the developmental, and their theories suffer accordingly in both explanatory power and appropriate clinical fit. Kernberg has lately acknowledged that the child-observation studies on separation-individuation do reinforce his clinical evidence (48).

Many other authors, lacking a specific developmental focus, search in vain for answers to these patients' problems in classical instinctual theory and oedipal conflict (see Chapter 13). It is *not* that the latter are not involved or important. It is that their importance *in these patients* must be subordinated to and perceived through the developmental focus of an arrested separation-individuation.

In the borderline patient specifically, this means that the therapist must be guided or oriented by what I have called the borderline triad: Separation-individuation leads to depression which leads to defense. Clinical observations about self- and object representations' instinctual-drive derivatives, ego functions and defense mechanisms, superego functions, fantasies, affective states, transference, and resistance must be organized around this essential theme. Again, this is not to say that other aspects are not important, but their importance must be subordinated to and organized around this theme.

Similarly, in the narcissistic patient, as described in Chapters 1 through 5, an understanding of the consequences of the separation-individuation failure is essential to conduct appropriate psychotherapy. This does not imply a whole new revolutionary metapsychology that discards the old but, rather, a new, additional perspective to add to those already in existence.

The major thrust of this book is to demonstrate the clinical effectiveness of this developmental approach with the narcissistic and borderline personality disorders.

PART I—THE PSYCHOPATHOLOGY OF NARCISSISM

Chapter 1, The Narcissistic Personality Disorder, describes the clinical picture, presents a developmental theory to explain that picture and then contrasts the theory with the theories of Kohut

(58-63) and Kernberg (43-50). Chapter 2, Differential Diagnosis, details the diagnostic differences (a) between the narcissistic personality disorder and the borderline disorder, (b) between both and the other major diagnostic categories, and (c) between both and the patient with a narcissistic defense against a borderline syndrome. Chapter 3 presents detailed case history and uses the clinical evidence to derive the intrapsychic structure of a patient with a narcissistic personality disorder. Chapters 4 and 5 describe in great detail the vicissitudes of that intrapsychic structure during the psychoanalytic psychotherapy of this patient. Chapter 4 presents the first or testing phase of treatment and Chapter 5 gives an interview-by-interview account of how the psychotherapeutic technique of interpretation of the patient's narcissistic vulnerability in the transference helps the patient to convert transference acting-out to therapeutic alliance and transference, which leads to a working-through of the underlying depression and fragmented self. Chapter 6 presents a new aspect of developmental theory: the narcissistic psychopathology (or psychopathology of the self) of the borderline patient and how it differs from that of the narcissistic personality disorder. It also describes the developmental theory and clinical picture of the borderline patient with a false self (117), contrasts this developmental view with that of Winnicott and then presents a detailed report of the psychoanalytic psychotherapy of two patients with a false self that illustrates the special technical treatment problems these patients present.

PART II—THE BORDERLINE PERSONALITY DISORDER

Chapter 7 presents a revision and update of the developmental theory of the roles of maternal libidinal availability and separation-individuation in normal ego development and in the developmental arrest of the borderline. This revision stems from reflection and study prompted by questions raised regarding the theory in the last eight years, as well as from a review of related studies published over the same period.

Chapter 8 puts the theory to the test by illustrating how the clinical evidence is used to determine the intrapsychic structure of three cases—one upper-level and two lower-level borderline patients.

Chapters 9 and 10, taken from previously published papers, have been extensively reworked and new cases have been added to demonstrate the treatment process of the three patients described in Chapter 8. Chapter 9 emphasizes the use of confrontation to establish a therapeutic alliance, while Chapter 10 focuses on the therapeutic techniques required to maintain the patient in the working-through phase of treatment. Chapter 11 describes the importance for successful treatment of the patient's mastery of the talionic impulse. Chapter 12 then presents problems involved in termination of treatment.

PART III—REFLECTIONS

Chapter 13 answers questions which have been raised about this developmental point of view; it then illustrates how misconceptions from opposite sides of the therapeutic spectrum—the psychoanalytic and the more directive therapies—can produce distortions in treatment of narcissistic and borderline patients. Finally, it recapitulates and summarizes the theme: Viewing the clinical evidence through the developmental perspective, specifically the vicissitudes and reverberations of the separation-individuation phase of ego development, leads to a unique and appropriate fit between theory and clinical evidence in patients with borderline and narcissistic personality disorders. This, in turn, leads to a more specific and effective treatment. The therapist who conducts treatment in this manner will discover that he or she has found the key to these disorders.

ACKNOWLEDGMENTS

I would like to thank Miss Helen Goodell for her usual superb job of editing, Mrs. Susan Barrows for some crucial suggestions about the manuscript, and my wife Pat for typing and preparing it.

I. The Psychopathology of Narcissism

The term "narcissism" has recently become so linked with one form of psychopathology that it is often overlooked that a normally developed or healthy narcissism, one definition of which is the libidinal investment of the self, is vital to a healthy adaptation. As originally described by Freud (25), the global infantile narcissism gradually differentiates with growth and maturation to invest the individual self-representation and provide the libidinal investment for the development of the capacities for regulating self-esteem, for self-assertion, for pursuit of one's own unique interests, for one's standards, ideals and ambitions.

This section presents the narcissistic personality disorder as one part of the wider spectrum of the psychopathology of narcissism: narcissistic defenses against an underlying borderline personality disorder and the narcissistic psychopathology of the borderline.

My interest in the narcissistic personality disorder has stemmed from and followed my work on the borderline syndrome (83, 86). From a superficial clinical point of view, these two disorders can be seen as opposite sides of the coin, with the borderline syndrome showing a deficient libidinal investment of the self, and the narcissistic personality disorder, on the surface at least, showing a grandiose and pathologically excessive libidinal investment of the self. This section makes clear how the psychopathology of narcissism differs in the two disorders. Kohut's failure to make this distinction has dramatized and greatly exaggerated the prevalence of the narcissistic personality disorder as a clinical problem. In my own clinical experience and that of many of my colleagues, as well as in the experience of hundreds of therapists across the country whom I have questioned, borderline patients far outnumber those with a narcissistic personality disorder in clinical practice.

Chapter 1 describes the clinical picture of the narcissistic personality disorder and then turns to developmental theory to account for that clinical picture. It thereby integrates the theoretical understanding of the narcissistic personality disorder with that of the borderline presented in prior publications and updated and elaborated in Chapters 7 to 12. These theoretical views are then contrasted with those of Kernberg (43-50) and Kohut (58-63). Chapter 2 on Differential Diagnosis furthers this integrated approach by emphasizing the same developmental theory to differentiate between the narcissistic personality disorder and the borderline personality disorder. It then devotes a special section to the presentation of a case illustrating a narcissistic defense against a borderline personality disorder; finally, it differentiates the two (narcissistic and borderline personality disorders) from other diagnostic categories such as psychosis, neurosis affective disorder, etc. Chapter 3 presents the case history of a narcissistic personality disorder and demonstrates how the clinical evidence is used to determine the intrapsychic structure. Chapters 4 and 5, presenting the psychoanalytic psychotherapy of this patient, demonstrate the

vicissitudes of the intrapsychic structure of the narcissistic personality disorder as they ebb and flow in response to the therapist's
interventions. Chapter 6 describes the narcissistic psychopathology
found in the borderline, gives an explanatory developmental
theory, contrasts this view with that of Winnicott (117) on the
false self and then presents two detailed illustrations of treatment
of borderline patients with a false self.

1

The Narcissistic
Personality Disorder

THE CLINICAL PICTURE

The main clinical characteristics of the narcissistic personality disorder are grandiosity, extreme self-involvement and lack of interest in and empathy for others, in spite of the pursuit of others to obtain admiration and approval. The patient manifesting a narcissistic personality disorder seems to be endlessly motivated to seek perfection in all he or she does, to pursue wealth, power and beauty and to find others who will mirror and admire his/her grandiosity. Underneath this defensive façade is a feeling state of emptiness and rage with a predominance of intense envy.

Three levels of functioning can be distinguished in the narcissistic disorders:

(a) Effective surface adaptation with success due to talent or skill. Such patients come for psychotherapy because of neurotic symptoms, sexual difficulty or difficulty in object relations.

(b) Patients with severe difficulty in object relations, usually along with neurotic symptoms and/or sexual problems.

(c) Those who function on a borderline level with ego weakness.

Meissner (90) describes four clinical types of narcissistic disorders:

1) phallic-narcissistic;
2) Nobel-prize narcissistic;
3) manipulatory or psychopathic;
4) needy, clinging and demanding.

To this list must be added what I call the "closet narcissist." Although, in a theoretical sense, all narcissists are closet narcissists, I am referring to the patient who presents him/herself as timid, shy, inhibited and ineffective—only to reveal later in therapy the most elaborate fantasies of the grandiose self.

The cases described below illustrate the clinical picture of the narcissistic disorder:

CASE ILLUSTRATIONS

Mr. X

Mr. X, 48, was married with two sons.

History of Present Illness

The patient came for treatment with the report that he had been one of the few men in line to be chosen as chief executive of a large corporation. Eagerly looking forward to this appointment, he was astounded and disappointed when called in by the board of directors and told that the appointment would go to his rival. He was even more astounded to learn the reason. The quality of his work was excellent, but his relationship with his employees and co-workers was so poor, that it made him ill-equipped to run the company.

Depressed and distraught, he returned home to seek support from his wife. To the contrary, she reinforced the observation of the board, saying he had the same problems with her and with their two children, with whom they had had considerable conflict; she added that he was for the most part quite self-involved and, although he could be quite stimulating and charming when he chose to be, usually he pursued his own interests and seemed quite unaware of either his wife's or his children's needs.

In the initial interview, as he came close to pointing out to me, the therapist, that obviously all of these people were mistaken, he checked himself and then reflected that there really must be something wrong with his perception, although he really couldn't see what it was. He had many complaints about his wife, her emotional inconsistency, coldness, needs and clinging. In the course of their 20 years of marriage, he had had a number of superficial affairs which rarely went beyond sexual liaisons.

He reported that both at work and with his family he felt he knew better how to manage situations and was quite devaluing and intolerant of their opinions. He smoked and drank heavily.

He complained further that he was not getting enough feedback from his wife, that "he was a sucker for women whom he admired and respected, who flattered him, and he expected such flattery and responded very positively to it. However, in his various affairs, after the early phase of sexual attraction and romance had run its course, he tended to lose interest and end one affair only to start another shortly afterwards.

He strove for perfection in his work and was intolerant of subordinates' failures to meet his standards, because it would reflect poorly on his own image. He was intolerant of any criticism and tended to lash out with anger without adequate thought or restraint. He had many outside interests: music, art, golf. The only neurotic symptom he reported was tension headaches; however, he reported an obsessive fear of and preoccupation with loneliness and death.

Past History

The patient was born in the West, the third of three children in a family which was serious, extremely religious and restrictive. He described being close to his father whom he liked, although the father was away from home a great deal when he was a child. The mother, he said, was much more punitive and restrictive than his father and administered all the discipline. There was very little pleasure in the home, since fun was not permitted, but emphasis was laid upon honor and duty. He was an outstanding student and athlete in high school and college, without any symptomatic episodes.

Evaluation

In the early sessions he demonstrated the following: Very early he began to have the same complaint about object relations with me that he had with his wife—"that there was not enough feedback"—when I did not ask a lot of questions. It was clear that on the one hand he idealized me and wished to call me by my first name, while on the other hand he tended to compete with me and devalue my various observations about him. This patient probably represents what has been described as the phallic, narcissistic character or as the most functional of the narcissistic disorders.

Mr. Y

The second patient is an example of the more common type of narcissistic disorder who comes for treatment with a middle level of functioning. The patient is a 36-year-old married man with two children, whose chief complaint is that he is in such a deep hole that he doesn't know how to get out of it other than by coming for treatment.

He was also stunned to hear from his wife that she was planning to divorce him and that she had felt it necessary to resort to a number of brief affairs over their 12-year marriage because of his self-centeredness and lack of involvement with her. He stated clearly that he was unable to be close to anyone, that he tended to pursue his own interests in a selfish manner, ignoring the needs of others, including his wife and children, until they confronted him with his egocentricity. Only then, in such a crisis atmosphere, would he become upset, change his behavior and attempt to conform to their wishes. He reported that they had had several of these crises in his marriage (although he hadn't known about his wife's affairs), and each time the crisis subsided he went back to his old habits. He said: "It seems that I have a need to be loved but cannot love; I am selfish; there is something horrible inside of me." He was deeply depressed, with vegetative signs. He was successful in his work as a businessman but had a number of sexual problems manifested by sexual acting-out. His memory of his childhood was sketchy, as he could recall very few of the events of those early developmental years.

Evaluation

This patient probably represents the middle range of narcissistic pathology, with extreme difficulty with object relations, neurotic symptomatology and sexual conflicts, although he is able to function quite well at work.

A DEVELOPMENTAL THEORY

Developmental theory sheds light on the developmental arrest and intrapsychic structure of the narcissistic personality disorder.

Level of Developmental Arrest of the Narcissistic Personality Disorder

It is a tenet of object relations theory (15, 16, 37, 38, 40, 41, 54, 55, 56, 57) that ego defense mechanisms and ego functions mature in parallel with the maturation of self- and object representations. A controversy has arisen over how to explain that the narcissistic personality disorder seems to violate this tenet in that a very primitive self-object representation is seen alongside a seemingly high capacity for ego functioning.

To put it in developmental terms, although the self-object representation is fused, the narcissistic personality disorder seems to get the benefit for ego development that is believed to come about only as a result of separation from that fusion. There has yet been no satisfactory resolution of this dilemma, either by myself (see below) or other authors (44, 63). We hope in the future to develop a theoretical postulate to resolve this ambiguity.

One of the functions of the rapprochement crisis during the separation-individuation phase of development is to bring into accord with reality by phase-appropriate disappointment and frustration those archaic structures, the grandiose self and the omnipotent object (76). Let us briefly review Mahler's observations on this isssue: Mahler noted that the chief characteristic of the practicing period is the child's great narcissistic investment in his or her own functions and his/her own body, as well as in the objects and objectives of his/her expanding "reality." He/she seems relatively impervious to knocks, falls and other frustrations.

The *rapprochement subphase* (15-22 months approximately) begins with the mastery of upright locomotion. Alongside the growth of the child's cognitive faculties and the increasing differentiation of his/her emotional life, there is also, however, a waning of his/her previous imperviousness to frustration, as well as of his/her relative obliviousness to the mother's presence.

An increased separation anxiety is observed: At the height of mastery, toward the end of the practicing period, there is increasingly clear differentiation between the self-representation and the object-representation. The toddler starts to lose his prior sense of grandiosity and omnipotence, and it begins to dawn on him that the world is not his oyster and that he must cope with it on his own.

The toddler returns to woo the mother, demanding that she share every aspect of his/her life, but it no longer works. The self-representation and the object representation are well on the way to differentiation. In this manner the infantile fantasies of grandiosity and omnipotence are brought into accord with reality.

The fixation of the narcissistic personality disorder must occur before this event because clinically the patient behaves as if the object representation were an integral part of the self-representation—an omnipotent, dual unity. The possibility of the existence of a rapprochement crisis doesn't seem to dawn on this patient. The fantasy persists that the world is his oyster and revolves about him. In order to protect this illusion, he must seal off by avoidance, denial and devaluation those perceptions of reality that do not fit or resonate with this narcissistic, grandiose self-projection. Consequently, he is compelled to suffer the cost to adaptation that is always involved when large segments of reality must be denied.

Why the fixation occurs at this level is a complex and poorly understood matter. Presumably, as with the borderline, the etiologic input can come from both sides of the nature-nurture spectrum. However, the input from both sides is much clearer in the borderline than in the narcissistic personality disorder.

Some of the mothers in narcissistic personality disorders are basically emotionally cold and exploitive. They ignore their children's separation-individuation needs in order to mold them into objects that will justify their own perfectionistic, emotional needs. The child's real individuation needs suffer as he or she resonates with the mother's idealizing projections. This identification with the mother's idealization leads to preservation of the grandiose self, which defends against the perception of the mother's failures and the child's associated depression.

A second possibility is suggested by the fact that in normal development the child, particularly the male, turns strongly in the early practicing phase, before rapprochement has occurred, to identify with the father. The child, experiencing an abandonment depression at the hands of the mother, could use this normal pathway as a vehicle or channel to "rescue" him/her from the abandonment depression and the mother. Rather than undergo the normal developmental process of identification with the father as a second, new, non-symbiotic object, the child transfers wholesale the symbiotic relationship with the mother onto the father in order to deal with his abandonment depression. The father thus becomes a target for projection of the symbiotic relationship with the mother. If the father is a narcissistic personality and this transfer occurs *before* the rapprochement phase, the child's grandiose self will still be preserved and reinforced through identification with the narcissistic father—thus producing a narcissistic disorder.

If the transfer occurs after the rapprochement phase has brought infantile grandiosity and omnipotence into accord with reality, the identification with the narcissistic disorder of the father will occur after the formation of the split object relations unit of the borderline, and a narcissistic defense against a borderline disorder will be superimposed on the underlying borderline intrapsychic structure (see pages 32-37). In other words, once the grandiose self has been brought into accord with reality during the rapprochement phase, it disappears and gives way to the separate split self- and object representations. Any turn to a narcissistic father after this event has taken place can only result in superimposing a later narcissistic identification on top of an underlying borderline intrapsychic structure.

This possibility raises some intriguing but so far unresolved developmental questions. It suggests that a narcissistic father may be essential for the production of a narcissistic defense against a borderline disorder. Since this turn to the father occurs earlier and more harmoniously in boys than in girls, it suggests that narcissistic disorders may be more common in boys than in girls, which seems to agree with clinical experience. Beyond that, the male child's rescue by the narcissistic father does not seem to lead commonly to homosexual problems, while the female child's rescue almost always leads to severe sexual conflicts during the oedipal period.

INTRAPSYCHIC STRUCTURE

Object Relations Fused-Units

The resultant intrapsychic structure of the narcissistic personality disorder from superficial clinical observation would appear to consist of only one object relations unit in contrast to the borderline's two part-units. It appears this way because of the unique continuous activation of the defensive unit while the other underlying unit only reveals itself in treatment as the continuity of the defenses is worked through.

The defensive or libidinal grandiose, self-omnipotent object relations fused-unit of the narcissistic personality disorder consists of an omnipotent fused object representation that contains all power, perfection, direction, supplies, etc. The grandiose self-representation is one of being superior, elite, exhibitionistic, with an affect of feeling perfect, special, unique. The projection of this defensive unit is so ubiquitous, global and airtight that it effectively conceals to the casual observer the underlying pathologic or aggressive fused-unit. When projecting the grandiose self, the patient exhibits his specialness and expects perfect mirroring of his grandiosity and unique perfection. When projecting the omnipotent object, he idealizes the perfection of the object which he expects to share; i.e., he shares and participates in the "narcissistic glow."

The underlying pathologic aggressive or empty object relations fused-unit consists of a fused object representation that is harsh, punitive and attacking and a self-representation of being humiliated, attacked, empty, linked by the affect of the abandonment depression. Kohut has called the self-representation of this fused-unit the fragmented self and organized his observations and theory around it. Kohut's work can be correlated with my own and with object relations theory in general if it is kept in mind that when Kohut refers to the fragmented self he is lumping together the entire aggressive or empty object relations fused-unit with the object representation, the abandonment depression and the self-representation.

Alliance Between the Defensive, Grandiose, Self-Omnipotent Object Fused-Unit and the Pathologic Ego

The defensive or grandiose object relations fused-unit forms an alliance with the pathologic ego to defend against the abandonment depression of the aggressive fused-unit, but this alliance operates in a different manner than that of the borderline. The abandonment depression of the aggressive fused-unit can be precipitated either by efforts at true self-activation, i.e., the pursuit of realistic self-expressive goals as opposed to the narcissistic goals of perfection, money, power, beauty, etc., or by the perception of the object's failure to provide perfect mirroring.

Alliance Between the Aggressive, Empty Object Relations Fused-Unit and the Pathologic Ego

This perception of the abandonment depression, if not immediately defended against by the defensive unit, activates an alliance between the aggressive unit and the pathologic ego in which the depression is dramatically externalized with a projection of its object representation as causing the depression, with massive denial of reality. The precipitation of the abandonment depression activates the alliance between the grandiose fused-unit and the pathologic ego, and the patient proceeds to avoid, deny and/or devalue the offending stimulus or perception, thereby restoring the balance of his narcissistic equilibrium and avoiding the experiencing of depression. The continuous, global projection of this defensive unit allows the narcissistic personality disorder to minimize the experience of depression and makes it appear that he gets his emotional supplies from within. In addition, the relatively free access to aggression enables the narcissistic personality disorder either to aggressively coerce the environment into resonating with his narcissistic projections or, if this fails, to deal with that failure by avoidance, denial and devaluation.

KOHUT ON THE NARCISSISTIC DISORDER AND THE PSYCHOLOGY OF THE SELF

Kohut's (58-63) unique contribution has been the observation of the vicissitudes of the clinical manifestations of images of the grandiose self and the omnipotent object, along with what he has called defects in the structure of the self.

Diagnosis and Clinical Picture

Kohut's view of diagnosis, however, has been more confusing than clarifying. He has defined the key pathology of the narcissistic disorder to be the primary defect in the structure of the self, not the clinical manifestations of grandiosity, exhibitionism, and narcissism. He, therefore, includes the types of disorders described by others (29, 30, 31, 35, 44, 83, 84, 86, 96, 97) as borderline under this concept and uses the term borderline to refer only to patients with borderline psychosis or schizophrenia. His clinical descriptions of some of the patients with narcissistic disorders closely resembled those of the borderline syndrome as described by myself and others. The affective states that Kohut described as fragmentation of the self, as well as defenses against it, seem quite similar to what I understand as the abandonment depression and its defense. It seems to me that there are cogent clinical and theoretical reasons for keeping the distinction between these two disorders clear and that Kohut's inclusive view of diagnosis has further confused an already confused area.

Kohut (63) described the defects in the structure of the self as being manifested clinically by defensive and compensatory structures beneath which lie low self-esteem, depression, a deep sense of uncared-for worthlessness and rejection, and a hunger for response and reassurance. I assume he is referring to a wide range of clinical phenomena similar to those I described as difficulties with self. These observations have broadened our clinical perception and given us tools to treat these patients. I found it fascinating, informed by Kohut's work, to observe the clinical manifestations of the grandiose self slowly emerge from behind the boulders of the patient's defenses.

I also agree with a number of Kohut's (63) other clinical impressions:

1) The differences in developmental level between the psychopathology of the self and the psychopathology of oedipal conflict.

2) His concept of the origin of excess aggression which differs

from that of Klein (57) and in certain respects from that of Kernberg (44). Kohut views normal aggression as vital to the evolution and self-assertive function of the self and feels that excess aggression is not inborn but comes from early trauma. Klein viewed it as inborn and Kernberg often refers to that notion as an etiological possibility in the borderline. It seems to me that, although it may sometimes be inborn, it more often in borderline and narcissistic patients comes from early trauma.

3) The need to pursue and recognize serious and latent, but denied, parental pathology.

Kohut's clinical observations of the psychopathology of the self have been widely accepted, but his theory of a psychology of the self has met with many objections (13, 47, 49, 100, 101, 110, 114). Some of these are due to his failure to clearly define his terminology. His writings seem to assume we know what he means by certain terms without adequately describing or defining them, for example: fragmentation of self, structure of the self, etc. Most objections, however, are to his view that narcissism has a separate line of development.

Kohut suggested that the self could be viewed from two complementary points of view: on the one hand, as the center of its own psychological universe; on the other, as part of the overall mental apparatus. He defined the self, in the former sense, as having its own functions—i.e., regulation of self-esteem through actualization of ambitions and ideals in reality. He saw the self as having its own development—aided by the mother's mirroring and the father's idealizing function—and its own psychopathology —structural defects related to failures in both mother's and father's functions.

This view, in my opinion, competes with, rather than complements, both object relations theory and the findings of child observation research and leads to conceptual confusions between the self and the object as part of the self, between the various stages or phases of the early development of the self- and object representation and finally between the differences in degree of psychological input into the developing self of the mother's mirroring function and the father's idealizing function. These theoretical confusions then lead to clinical confusions about the nature of the transference and what level of emotional conflict is being worked through in the treatment.

The Bipolar Self

In emphasizing the need for a psychology of the self, Kohut (63) makes a cogent argument that drive experience is subordinated to the child's experience of self and, as he puts it, self-objects. It seems to me that this is an argument for the use of an object relations theory of development. However, he stresses, instead, narcissism as a separate line of development of the bipolar self and it is this issue which has raised the greatest objections.

He joins the object to the self, i.e., objects are self-objects, thereby creating a separate line of development via this concept of self-objects at the cost of considerable confusion, semantic and otherwise, of self and object as part of the self. Furthermore, this concept, which implies that there is no separation of self from object, but rather growth and maturation from archaic to more mature forms, does away with the need for phases of development (symbiosis and separation-individuation) and for separation of the self from the object.

It seemingly excludes object relations altogether, leading to the possibility of a therapy that concentrates so exclusively on repairing the patient's narcissistic wounds that its end product could be a patient whose narcissistic defect is repaired and who is able to autonomously regulate self-esteem and articulate wishes in reality, but whose object relations continue on a narcissistic level.

The evidence of child observation (76) research tends to confirm the reciprocal interrelatedness of the development of the self and of object relations as outlined by Freud (24, 25) in his early papers and as recently reemphasized by Kernberg (47) and Giovacchini (35)—i.e., "Object relations can be traced back to their narcissistic precursors. The latter make development possible and, in turn, continue to develop" (35). In other words, it confirms the idea of separation of self from the object, and it contradicts the notion of the perpetuation of self-objects. This is further confirmed by the following clinical experiences with borderline and narcissistic patients in analytic therapy: Patients who are working through their abandonment depression or separation of the self from the maternal object report that the mother's withdrawal is experienced as a loss of a vital part of the self, thus relating self to object. When patients whose principal defense is clinging to the object improve, one observes a slow, gradual decrease in the cathexis of the object representation, simultaneously with a parallel slow and gradual increase in the cathexis of the self-representation. Although there may, admittedly, be other explanations, the most likely is that the emotional investment is being transferred from the object representation to the self-representation, thereby providing further evidence that self and object are initially linked and then separate. This separation is followed by progressive, separate, parallel maturation of both self- and object representations, mutually influencing each other.

Kohut's ignoring of this transfer of investment and consequent maturation leads to confusion as to the relative degree of influence of the mother and the father on the child's developing self-representations as well as to confusion about the phase of influence of each parent. Kohut seemingly equates the influence of the mother's mirroring function on the grandiose self between the ages of one and three with the father's idealizing influence on the idealized parent image between the ages of four and six:

> If the mother had failed to establish a firmly cohesive self in the child, the father may yet succeed in doing so. If the exhibitionistic component of the nuclear self cannot become consolidated, then its voyeuristic component may yet give it form and structure (63, p. 9).

An argument could be made for this point of view in normal development, where the child individuates and separates from the mother and therefore becomes more intrapsychically available for the full input of the father. However, the child's relationship with the father is then mediated through a separate self-representation in a triadic intrapsychic structure, rather than a fused symbiotic self-object representation in a dyadic structure. What then is to be understood by Kohut's notion of a merger or twinship with the father that implies symbiotic ties that, according to object relations theory, would have been already resolved?

Beyond that, in pathological arrests such as narcissistic and borderline disorders, where the child has not separated from the mother and is therefore not fully available for the input by the father, it seems to me that there is questionable validity to the notion that mother's and father's influences can be equated or, for that matter, that father's idealizing function can adequately compensate for the mother's defects in mirroring. In other words, in early development, the child first learns to feel his/her own unique, individual thoughts, wishes, and strivings mediated by the mother's mirroring. He/she learns to feel entitled to these strivings and to have support for them; only after the child has made them his/her own in this fashion can he/she go on to shape them into reality through ideals. If the former function, which derives from the mother, remains impaired, it has to also impair the latter function. It seems to me that an idea possibly applicable to the normal developmental process is inappropriately applied to a pathological arrest.

The ignoring of phases and equating of mother's mirroring and father's idealizing impel Kohut in his evaluation of clinical conditions, as illustrated in all three case reports in his book (63), to the view that the identification with father compensated for the deficiencies with mother and formed the basis of a transference that allowed the working-through of the conflict with the father and therefore the freeing of the compensatory mechanisms without having to work out the conflict with mother.

My own point of view is that the patients he described have transferred what I would call their clinging symbiotic transference from the mother to the father, who was then in the intrapsychic sense not a father in his own right but mainly a symbol for the mother. Therefore, in treatment the mirroring and idealizing conflicts are worked through vis-à-vis the mother, not the father. The intrapsychic structure and the transference remain dyadic, not triadic.

Beyond that, it seems to me that Kohut's view could lead to such an emphasis on repair of compensatory mechanisms that adequate attention might not be paid to working-through the conflict with the mother, which could lead in some cases to settling for less than optimum results.

The Mother's Defective Mirroring

The early mother-child interaction is so complex, yet so fateful for a child's development, that it is both difficult and hazardous to try to tease out principal, generalizable themes. Nevertheless, the stereotyped repetition of these maladaptive themes in our patients' lives and in the transference impels us to undertake this task in spite of its hazards, in hopes of unraveling some of its mysteries. This is acceptable as long as we keep in mind the limitations. It is essential, if we are to understand our patients' problems and their therapeutic needs.

There seems to me to be some ambiguity in Kohut's comments about the role of the mother. At one point he emphasizes that mothers are often sicker than their superficial appearances would suggest, which certainly reflects my own clinical experience. However, his conception of why and how the mother's mirroring function is defective seems to me to describe only part of the picture. He describes the mother as lacking empathy for the child's grandiose exhibitionistic self. In other words, she is not able to understand or respond for a variety of possible reasons, none of which seem to have anything specifically to do with that child. The reasons may be her narcissism, her depression, her psychotic state, etc. Although this is no doubt true in some cases, far more often in my experience the mother's defective mirroring springs from a specific emotional withdrawal, because this specific child is expressing his/her own unique self or grandiose exhibitionistic self. This self-expression interrupts or frustrates his/her resonating with the projections the mother had placed on the child in order to shape him or her for use as an object essential to maintain her own intrapsychic equilibrium. More importantly, it seems to me, Kohut overlooks the profound effects of the other part of this theme, the mother's reward for those regressive behaviors that fulfill her projections, thereby gratifying her clinging and relieving her anxiety. This theme is overlooked, despite the fact that it is described a number of times (63):

> . . . The mother's empathy, one might assume, was not lacking altogether—it was faulty, rather than flat; when he injured himself, she had, after all, responded—and it did occasionally confirm his sense of his worthwhileness, and thus of the reality of his self (p. 9).

> . . . On innumerable occasions she appeared to have been totally absorbed in the child—overcaressing him, completely in tune with every nuance of his needs and wishes—only to withdraw from him suddenly, either by turning her attention totally to other interests or by grossly and grotesquely misunderstanding his needs and wishes (p. 55).

> . . . Were I formulating my interpretation of her today, I would say that positive mirroring responses from the environment would be forthcoming only if she could first relieve her mother's depression. Her depressions were therefore partly the reenactment of her deep sense of failure vis-à-vis this demand from her depressed mother. Or, seen from a slightly different viewpoint, she was convinced that the maternal selfobject would not provide her with self-esteem, enhancing acceptance and approval, unless she, the small child, could first fulfill the mother's similar needs (pp. 60-61).

This denial reached its height in his argument against a disorder of the self resulting from instinctual fixation or oral fixation points, with corresponding developmental arrest of the ego as the result of "addiction to infantile gratification" (63, p. 73). It is not addiction to infantile gratification as such but the push-pull of reward for regression and withdrawal for separation-individuation.

In other words, the emotional state of being cared for, being fed, induced by the infantile gratification, stands in dramatic contrast to the stark affective experience of abandonment depression.

In his argument against such a possibility, Kohut states that it could only be brought about by parents who indulged pregenital drives and blocked the child's phallic genital needs: "I don't believe such a decisive blocking could be carried out even by parents who are in minimal empathic contact with the maturational aspirations of their child" (63, p. 73). In this statement, the author denies that the mother's responses do indeed block not only phallic-genital needs, but also and more importantly, the primitive and fundamental need for individuation—to be a separate, autonomously functioning individual.

KERNBERG ON THE NARCISSISTIC PERSONALITY DISORDER

Kernberg (44, 47, 49) holds that the narcissistic personality is not due to a developmental arrest or fixation at early narcissistic stages of development; rather, it is due to simultaneous development of pathological forms of self-love and of pathological forms of object-love. He begins with Jacobson's (40, 41) notion that in early development, after self- and object-images are differentiated and ego boundaries and reality-testing have developed, extreme frustration can cause a regression of self- and object-images and the loss of reality-testing and a psychotic regression. He then proposes that in the narcissistic personality there is a refusion of self- and object-images at a point in development when ego boundaries have become stable. There follows a fusion of ideal self, ideal object, and actual self-images without destruction of object-images.

This "regressive refusion" theory violates a fundamental tenet of object relations theory and raises questions that have yet to be answered; ego development moves parallel, both forward and regressively backward, with the development of self- and object representations. In fact, some believe that the former is responsible for the development of the latter. Jacobson honors this tenet, since, as self- and object representations regress, so does ego development, and the patient becomes psychotic. Kernberg now proposes that, in the narcissistic personality, self- and object representations regressively refuse without causing a regression in ego development, something which heretofore was not believed to be possible.

Furthermore, Kernberg attempts to buttress his argument that the narcissistic personality is not a developmental arrest by comparing the features of the narcissistic personality with what he describes as "normal narcissism of small children." For example, according to Kernberg (44), the following features distinguish pathological narcissism from the normal narcissism of small children:

1) The grandiose fantasies of normal small children, their angry efforts to control mother and to keep themselves in the center of everybody's attention, have by far a more realistic quality than is the case of narcissistic personalities.

2) Small children's overreaction to criticism, failure, and blame, as well as their need to be the center of attention, admiration and love, coexists with simultaneous expression of genuine love and gratitude, interest in their objects at times when they are not frustrated, and, above all, with the capacity to trust and depend upon significant objects. A two-and-a-half-year-old child's capacity to maintain a libidinal investment in mother during temporary separations is in striking contrast to the narcissistic patient's inability to depend upon other people (including the analyst) beyond immediate need gratification.

3) Normal infantile narcissism is reflected in the child's demandingness related to real needs, while the demandingness of pathological narcissism is excessive, cannot ever be fulfilled, and regularly reveals itself to be secondary to a process of internal destruction of the supplies received.

4) The coldness and aloofness of patients with pathological narcissism at times when their capacity for social charm is not in operation, their tendency to disregard others except when temporarily idealizing them as potential sources of

narcissistic supply, and the contempt and devaluation prev-
alent in most of their relationships are in striking contrast
to the warm quality of the small child's self-centeredness.
Pursuing this observation into the historical analysis of narcissistic patients, one finds from the age of two to three years
a lack of normal warmth and engagement with others, and
an easily activated, normal destructiveness and ruthlessness.

This argument, it seems to me, falls by its own weight, as it
ignores the developmental implications of the work of both
Mahler (76) and Bowlby (7, 8). One cannot compare the clinical
manifestation of a developmental arrest with that of normal development and then argue that these differences indicate that the
former cannot be an arrest of the latter, because it is the arrest that
produces the differences. This issue is strikingly clear in example
#2, where Kernberg argues that the two-and-one-half-year-old's
capacity to maintain a libidinal investment in mother during
separation is in striking contrast to the narcissistic patient's inability to depend upon other people. Of course it is, because the
narcissistic patient's developmental arrest occurs probably long
before two and one half years, when this capacity develops. The
effects of the rapprochement crisis in deflating narcissism are
ignored. Beyond that, why should one think that the consequences
to the early development of the child of interactions with a normal
mother should resemble those with a pathologic mother?

My own point of view is that the narcissistic personality disorder
is a developmental arrest, since in treatment the patient's abandonment depression or fragmentation of the self can be precipitated either by narcissistic disappointment at the hands of the
object or by his own efforts towards self-expression or self-in-
dividuation. It is this latter that suggests a true developmental
arrest of individuation has occurred.

Although he disagrees about the origin of the narcissistic personality as described above, Kernberg accepts, as do most others,
Kohut's description of the clinical manifestation of the narcissistic
personality. However, he again disagrees with Kohut's therapeutic

approach of "accepting the admiration" of the "developing idealizing transference," feeling that this approach neglects the intimate relationship between narcissistic and object-related conflicts and the crucial conflicts regarding aggression and may unwittingly foster an interference with the full development of the negative transference. In contrast, Kernberg argues for a systematic analysis of the positive and negative aspects of the patient's grandiosity from an essentially neutral position.

Although I disagree with Kernberg's view of the origins of the narcissistic personality, I share his view of the clinical picture and his psychotherapeutic approach with the reservation that the "systematic analysis" of the negative transference emphasizes the interpretation of the patient's exquisite need for perfect mirroring or idealizing and his profound disappointment and rage when this need is frustrated by the reality of the therapist. As mentioned, I also think it important to analyze the abandonment depression that occurs as the patient attempts separation-individuation.

The next chapter on Differential Diagnosis emphasizes the differences between the narcissistic personality disorder and the borderline as a prelude to presenting the different treatment techniques required by the two disorders.

2

Differential
Diagnosis

The narcissistic and borderline personality disorders must be distinguished first from each other and then from psychoses, affective disorders and psychopathic personality.*

NARCISSISTIC PERSONALITY DISORDER VERSUS BORDERLINE PERSONALITY DISORDER

The two disorders can be distinguished by developmental level, intrapsychic structure, clinical manifestations, and transference, as well as by the psychotherapeutic technique required for treatment.

---

* The reader may question why DSM III (2a) is not referred to in this chapter. The clinical description of the narcissistic disorder used here is the same as in DSM III. In my view, the clinical description of the borderline syndrome used here not only includes all of the DSM III criteria, but is also far more comprehensive and specific.

Developmental Level

The narcissistic personality disorder must be fixated or arrested before the developmental level of the rapprochement crisis, since one of the important tasks of that crisis is not performed, i.e., the deflation of infantile grandosity and omnipotence. The intrapsychic structure of the narcissistic personality disorder preserves the infantile grandiosity and narcissistic link to the omnipotent object.

The rapprochement crisis, on the other hand, is crucial to the borderline, whose pathology can be seen as a reflection of his/her immersion in and inability to resolve it. Clinically, he behaves as if all life were one long, unresolvable rapprochement crisis.

Intrapsychic Structure

As described in Chapter 1, the intrapsychic structure of the narcissistic personality disorder consists of a grandiose self-representation and omnipotent object-representation which have fused into one unit which is more or less continuously activated to defend against the underlying aggressive or empty object relations fused-unit. This continuous activation minimizes the experiencing of depression.

This narcissistic style of defense differs from the borderline's, where the self- and object representations are not fused but separate and split into rewarding and withdrawing part-units. The projections of these two part-units are not continuous but alternating. They call for passive-regressive behavior which requires the forgoing of the true self and self-assertion. The borderline patient then does not have as free access to aggression as does the narcissistic personality disorder. Thus, self-assertion, coming up against the maternal withdrawal projection, is not available for self-esteem. The borderline defends by clinging to or distancing from the object.

The borderline's projections of the rewarding and withdrawing units are not so global, airtight, or intense that reality events have to be totally denied, devalued or avoided. Unlike the narcissistic patient, the borderline is hypersensitive to reality, particularly to people's rewarding and withdrawing responses. The borderline perceives the reality as inducing depression and then clings to or distances from the object for relief, meanwhile denying the destructiveness of these defenses to adaptation.

Clinical Manifestations and Transference Acting-out

The differences in developmental level and intrapsychic structure are seen clinically most clearly in the transference acting-out. The continuity of the self-representation of the narcissistic disorder in treatment presents a seemingly invulnerable armor of grandiosity, self-centeredness, exhibitionism, arrogance and devaluation of others. These characteristics are in marked contrast to the self-representation of the borderline, which alternates between brittle, vulnerable, self-depreciative, clinging behavior and erratic and irrational outbursts of rage.

The depression beneath the narcissistic personality disorder's defenses is heavily colored with narcissistic outrage and feelings of humiliation. The rage has a quality of "coldness" or lack of relatedness. In contrast, the borderline patient's depression is dominated by feelings of inadequacy about and hostility toward the self, and the rage shows intense relatedness. The themes of pursuit of power and perfection, wealth and beauty so prominent in the narcissist are at best minor in the borderline. Envy in the borderline is subordinated to depression and anger at the loss of wished-for supplies, while it is a prominent theme in the narcissist. Although all patients come to treatment with mixed motives, a predominant share of the narcissistic personality disorder's motivations is to find and fulfill the perfection he seeks, as well as to have the therapist provide the adulation and perfect mirroring he hungers for. The key word here is *perfect,* for it contrasts so markedly with the borderline patient, who seeks not perfect mirroring of his grandiosity but bare acknowledgment of the existence of his self-representation as well as fulfillment of his fantasy of receiving supplies.

Although the psychotherapy of the narcissistic personality disorder will be presented in detail in Chapters 4 and 5, a brief explanation is presented here to emphasize the differences in psychotherapeutic technique between the two disorders.

Therapeutic Technique

The consequences of the idealizing and mirroring projections of the narcissistic patient and the regressive projections of the borderline patient help to explain why the therapeutic techniques used with these disorders—confrontation with the borderline, interpretation with the narcissistic disorder—are not reciprocally effective.

One must confront the narcissistic patient not with behavior which is destructive to himself, for with his grandiose self-image he is not able to perceive that fact; rather one must point out aspects of reality which he is denying, devaluing or avoiding, since the grandiose self does not perceive the harm done either to his object relations or to his eventual true self-interests. The confrontation of the harmfulness of the behavior in reality is experienced as an attack and has to be defended against by denial, devaluation or avoidance, as was the original reality incident. Consequently, therapeutic technique emphasizes interpretation of the patient's vulnerability to narcissistic disappointment of his grandiosity and need for perfection as seen in the transference acting-out.

In contrast, the borderline who is denying that his defensive behavior is destructive to the self reacts to the confrontation or the bringing of this fact to his attention not as an attack from without, but as a constructive therapeutic effort which he integrates in order not to be any more harmful to himself than necessary.

Beyond that, if the therapeutic technique so useful with the narcissistic disorder is employed too early with the borderline, it forecloses the development of a therapeutic alliance, placing the therapist in the position of reinforcing the rewarding unit and fostering transference acting-out of the rewarding part-unit/pathologic-ego alliance.

A clinical vignette illustrates the differences between confrontation and interpretation with the borderline patient.

A young woman is hospitalized and calls to tell her mother she is in a mental hospital. The mother hears her daughter but ignores this information to scapegoat the daughter, telling her that her brother is drinking again and that she, the patient, must speak to him about it. The patient reports this incident with an affect of dismay and disappointment.

> *Interpretation* (Kohut (63)): Even though these interactions with your mother are disappointing, you seem compelled to seek them out in order to feel good about yourself.

> *Confrontation* (Masterson (83, 86)): Since these interactions disappoint you or are painful to you, why do you seek your mother out at these times? Why do you let your mother treat you this way?

The interpretation suggests why the patient behaves as she does, while the confrontation brings to her attention how destructive the behavior is to herself and invites her to investigate why. The answer to this question then comes from the patient, not the therapist, thus avoiding the possibility that the patient might use the therapist's interpretation not for insight but for resistance and transference acting-out.

NARCISSISTIC DEFENSE AGAINST A BORDERLINE DISORDER

Differentiation of the two disorders is further complicated by the fact that some borderline patients develop a narcissistic defense against their borderline problem. This may result, as mentioned previously, from a child who is experiencing an abandonment depression at the hands of his/her mother turning to a narcissistic father for "rescue" after the rapprochement phase has deflated infantile grandiosity and omnipotence. The narcissistic defense initially present may confuse the therapist's diagnosis unless he is careful to observe the borderline intrapsychic structure emerge as the narcissistic defense is worked through. On the other hand, if the patient begins treatment in a regressed state, the borderline disorder may be observed first and the narcissistic defense will only emerge later in psychotherapy. This does not indicate a change in diagnosis but a change in defense.

Ann B.

When first seen, this young woman was clearly in a regressed borderline state. As the psychotherapy progressed, rather than move into working-through of her conflict with the mother (borderline conflict), the patient moved into a full-fledged narcissistic defense against this conflict, which took several years to work through, before she returned to working-through the underlying conflict with the mother. The intricate and complex linkages between the narcissistic defense and the borderline conflict, as well as their relationship with later oedipal condensations, will be shown as they emerged in psychotherapy in Chapters 9 and 10. It suffices here for the purpose of differential diagnosis to present the history.

The patient illustrated the narcissistic defense against the borderline problem by describing that she had two selves: a self that was dependent, needy, helpless and clinging and a self that was superior, cool, in control but had very little affect. Under separation stress she would regress from the father self to the mother self, which she described as being like "falling through the roof" into helplessness, i.e., she had no firm foundation to her self-image. The history indicates the presence of the borderline problem in her symptomatic episodes and the narcissistic defense in her high-level functioning at school in between these episodes.

History of Present Illness

Ann B., 21, recently graduated from college with honors, moved to New York City to live on her own and start her first job. This separation stress brought on attacks of panic: "The terror just swept over me. I was afraid that my legs wouldn't work or that I wouldn't be able to eat or swallow. I thought perhaps I was going crazy." In addition, she complained of hysterical episodes of impaired consciousness and recurrent depressions. Associated with these episodes of panic were feelings of helplessness and inability to cope. She became obsessed "with what might happen if the fear took over." Clearly the borderline problem and her mother-self had the upper hand at that moment.

She reported previous episodes of depression on the first day of summer camp at age nine, in the twelfth grade in high school, and during the first year of college. She reiterated her lack of confidence in herself in this state and her enormous feeling of dependence on her mother. She reported that whenever she got panicky she would call her mother for reassurance, sometimes several times in a day. She currently had a boyfriend whom she idealized and to whom she clung.

Family History

She described her mother as being phobic and excessively preoccupied with the home and family. At the beginning of psychotherapy she emphasized that the mother rewarded her infantile behavior; later she reported that the mother vigorously attacked any of her efforts at self-assertiveness or originality. The mother attacked her for her body shape, her body functions, and, eventually, her emerging sexuality, finding all of it "disgusting." The father, on the other hand, giving a hint of the narcissistic defense, was described as very successful, extremely self-centered, and narcissistic. He showed little affect and patronized and looked down upon his wife but actively sought out and indulged both of his children, particularly the patient. She had one younger sister who was phobic. When the patient was between eight and ten years of age, severe conflict developed between mother and father, with the father being suspected of having a number of extramarital affairs. This conflict between mother and father drove the patient even closer to the father, and she became his favorite and constant companion, participating in many activities with him without the mother. The narcissistic defense was by now becoming institutionalized and was in charge.

Associated with this growing closeness to her father, attacks of separation anxiety in the form of anxiety and nausea before going to school in kindergarten gradually subsided as the narcissistic defense took over, and she functioned extremely well in grammar and high school, getting straight A's. Despite this high level of functioning, when physically ill she would become extremely anxious. In the twelfth grade she was depressed for about six months; this ended when she met her first boyfriend.

Although she feared she might become depressed if she attended college away from home, she went anyway and initially did become extremely depressed, cried, and called home almost every day for most of the first year. However, the narcissistic defense again took over, and she adapted well for the next three years, graduated with honors, and moved to the city to look for a job.

She dated one boy throughout twelfth grade, having mostly an intellectual relationship: "He needed me more than I needed him." During college she dated another boy for a few years and had intercourse for the first time without difficulty. She was currently dating exclusively a man she described as gentle, caring and upright, the family's idea of the perfect mate.

Intrapsychic Structure

The patient had a basic underlying borderline intrapsychic structure that consisted of the following: A rewarding maternal part-object representation that was of an omnipotent, god-like mother who provided safety and the associated affect of relief from panic and anxiety and "feeling good and loved." The part-self-image was that of a helpless and compliant child. The withdrawing maternal part-object representation was that of an extremely angry, attacking and punitive and vengeful mother who found her disgusting in her essence, i.e., her individuation, and who would kill her. The associated affect was compounded principally of fear, rage and depression. The part-self image was of being guilty, an insect, a worm, worthless, despicably bad and inadequate because she was a woman, like the mother.

The pathological ego functioned to maintain the wish for reunion and abet the fulfillment of the mother's wishes by avoiding separation, self-assertion and individuation, behaving in a helpless, dependent, unassertive, clinging, needy and asexual manner, meanwhile denying the destructiveness of this behavior to her adaptation.

Whenever she was exposed to separation trauma, i.e., mother's withdrawal or its symbol, she would collapse in helpless, fearful, hysterical panic which, from the history, was designed to coerce the withdrawing mother to return and "take care of her," which in real life she actually did. The patient referred to this part of her self-image associated with the borderline conflict and the mother as "her mother-self."

The Narcissistic Defense

As an effort to resolve this dilemma with her mother and to get revenge, and aided by the father's seductive behavior, she turned from the mother to the father—again probably after rapprochement had deflated her infantile grandiosity—and made an intense identification with his narcissistic character structure, which then produced an overlay of narcissistic defense against the borderline conflict.

In this narcissistic intrapsychic structure, the object representation was omnipotent, controlling, all-powerful, the self-representation being grandiose and special, the affect being that of feelings of superiority, uniqueness and well-being based on the acting-out of this unit, through narcissistically manipulating other people to obtain their approval, devaluing them and using them solely for this narcissistic purpose and also being able to act without sexual feeling, i.e., to use sex as a manipulation for her narcissistic need. This self part-representation the patient described as "her father-self," which was cool, superior, affectless.

Phallic Oedipal Stage

The identification with the narcissistic father in the latter part of the separation-individuation phase apparently "rescued" the patient from the intense borderline conflict with the mother at the cost of severe conflict in the oedipal stage. The patient colluded with the father's seduction to get revenge on the mother by taking the father away from her and thereby developed a pattern of sexual acting-out. The fact that the relationship was so actively acted out though not in an overt sexual manner then stirred up her oedipal wishes. She developed intense guilt regarding acting out the revenge on the mother, which then was secondarily condensed with guilt regarding her oedipal feelings with the father. The mother's original disparaging of her emerging sexuality combined with the oedipal sources of guilt to produce a feminine self-image of being profoundly bad, revengeful, unworthy and guilty and not deserving of a real relationship with a man.

Under separation stress, the shift would take place from the father-self to the mother-self, which she described as "falling through the roof of her personality, going from being cool, detached, superior and in control (father-self) to being helpless, needy and clinging (mother-self).

The patient began treatment in this regressed state as a result of her separation panic so that it was necessary to begin the work with this conflict. As she began to form a transference and resolve some of the conflict, she moved in treatment, as she had as a child, from the borderline conflict to the narcissistic identification with the father and her father-self. It then became necessary to work through the narcissistic defense as well as its phallic-oedipal condensations in full before finally and fully returning to the borderline conflict. These details are described in Chapters 9 and 10.

UPPER-LEVEL VERSUS LOWER-LEVEL BORDERLINE

The higher- and middle-level narcissistic personality disorders have been described in Chapter 1, and the lower-level is discussed later in this chapter as psychopathic personality. Differences between higher- and lower-level borderlines are presented here. The upper-level borderline's clinical picture is most often neurotic-like. Although he has the twin fears of abandonment or engulfment, his principal fear is abandonment, and his principal form of defense is clinging, not distancing. The reverse can be said of the lower-level borderline, who also has fears of both engulfment and abandonment but whose principal fear by far is that of engulfment and whose principal defense is distancing. The lower-level patient is prone to temporary psychotic attacks under separation stress, as well as to feelings of depersonalization, unreality and paranoid projections.

The therapeutic prognosis is better for the upper-level border-line than for the lower-level borderline. In the section on treatment, one upper-level and two lower-level borderlines will be presented. In order to emphasize the clinical picture of the lower-level borderline, to which I have perhaps not given adequate attention before, two brief case illustrations are described below.

Case 1

A 17-year-old girl was admitted to the hospital with a three-year history of drug abuse, excessive use of alcohol, and excessive weight loss. She was having difficulty with a boyfriend and her parents were getting a divorce. Recently she had developed feelings of panic, with sweating, palpitations and an acute sense of fear, as well as depression; finally, she made a suicide attempt, which precipitated admission.

The family history was positive in that the maternal grandmother had been hospitalized with similar symptoms, and the patient's father had had a nervous breakdown. On examination, there was no thinking disorder, her affect was shallow and she reported feelings of depersonalization and unreality, in addition to her depression and panic. At one point she felt the floor moving up towards her and at another time she felt her thigh shaking and changing its shape.

Three months after hospitalization, she experienced an acute psychotic decompensation with paranoid ideation and hallucinatory experiences. The decompensations would respond to Mellaril over a number of weeks and then recur, usually under therapeutic pressure. After a number of months the psychotic decompensations disappeared and were replaced by acute behavioral disturbances—putting her fist through windows, breaking light bulbs and scratching—as she moved into an acute suicidal phase. These cycles of psychotic episodes followed by behavioral disturbance followed by improvement kept recurring; every time she was up for discharge and apparently ready to leave the hospital, a psychotic disorganization would ensue.

Case 2

A 34-year-old woman was seen in consultation for her failure to improve over five years of psychotherapy. She gave an early history of marginally successful adaptation throughout her younger life and graduation from high school. However, beginning shortly after graduation from high school, in close association with her father's terminal illness, she was for several years a day patient in the state hospital. Since then she had never returned to an adequate level of functioning.

There were times when her behavior was so out of control that hospitalization was almost indicated for control. There were also times when the level of distortion in the interpersonal processes reached the point of being psychotic. She worked at a clerical job, led a sheltered life, living at home with her mother and sister, and felt intruded upon by this sister and her two children. She had been tried on a variety of medications without much success except that they seemed to prevent her social withdrawal and deterioration.

On examination she complained that she had a feeling that "nothing is real for the last 14 years," that she had constant nightmares, and feelings of unreality and depersonalization. She was also observed to have paranoid projections.

She continued: "I have to force myself to function every day to go to work. Once I went into the hospital, it was very hard to leave. I can do my work, because all I do is file workmen's compensation claims, and I am isolated from relationships with people. I have to force myself not to jump from open windows or out of cars or not to slit my wrists. It is a daily temptation. I feel dead but have to keep going." The patient spoke of herself as a "she," a "her," or "that thing." Outside of functioning at work, the patient sat in her chair at home and did nothing.

It is significant and typical of borderline patients that despite the serious illness she showed as an adult, her childhood history was seemingly quite benign. She was protected by the dependency umbrella of childhood, and it took the stress of adult responsibility to expose her vulnerability. For 12 years she went to a local parochial school, where she was a good student. She worked hard, was viewed as being "very quiet" and interested in music. She wanted to be a singer and sang in the choir and in the local community theater as a teenager. Her graduation from high school was "the beginning of the end. I didn't know what I would do."

DIFFERENTIATION OF NARCISSISTIC AND BORDERLINE DISORDERS FROM OTHER MENTAL ILLNESS

This section differentiates both the narcissistic personality disorder and the borderline personality disorder from psychosis, affective disorder, psychopathic personality, and neurosis.

Differentiation of Both Disorders from Psychosis

This is more of an issue with the borderline because of the presence, particularly in the lower-level borderline, of transient though reversible psychotic-like episodes, the tendency to primary process thinking, paranoid projections, and feelings of depersonalization and unreality. The two latter symptoms—paranoid projections and feelings of depersonalization and unreality—may be present in a narcissistic personality disorder, which then must also be differentiated from psychosis, principally schizophrenia.

The intrapsychic structure of the schizophrenic reveals a fused self-object representation, poor ego boundaries and poor reality-testing, which is persistent and not reversible. In contrast, the borderline has separate split self- and object images which are consistent, stronger ego boundaries, and better reality-testing. The narcissistic personality disorder, although he or she has fused self-object representation, has the firmest ego boundaries of all three and the best reality perception, except where his narcissistic projections are involved.

These intrapsychic features of the schizophrenic and borderline reflect pathologic fixations at the symbiotic and separation-individuation levels of development and suggest that those schizophrenics with a psychodynamic etiology are the developmental neighbors of the borderline. The borderline separates from the symbiotic relationship with the mother and gets the dividends of that separation, i.e., stronger ego boundaries, defenses and functions, at the cost of an abandonment depression. The patient with schizophrenia, however, is unable to separate and remains fixated in the symbiotic stage, for which he or she pays the price of weaker ego boundaries, defenses and functions. The fused self-object representation that results from fixation at the symbiotic stage can, on casual clinical observation, appear to be similar to the borderline clinging relationship with the maternal part-object. However, careful observation will usually reveal that the schizophrenic describes a fused self-object representation, not separate split self- and object representations. In addition, the psychotic episodes of the borderline usually occur under separation stress and usually abate when the separation stress is relieved. This has an important clinical consideration: If the borderline patient is hospitalized, antipsychotic drugs should not be prescribed until enough time has elapsed to determine if the episode will subside because of hospitalization alone. On the other hand, in unstable cases the administering of an antipsychotic drug can be almost a diagnostic test, in that borderline patients often do not respond well to antipsychotics (particularly chlorpromazine and its derivatives), so that if the psychosis responds and the patient's thinking clears up, it is a strong indication that he or she may be schizophrenic.

Differentiation of Both Disorders from Affective Disorder

This differentiation applies more to the borderline than to the narcissistic personality disorder. The discovery of the therapeutic effect of lithium has brought about a remarkable resurgence of interest in manic-depressive disorders. One of the handicaps of this resurgence is a tendency to overdiagnose the condition, since we now have a therapy for it. This resurgence has also led some investigators to look further afield to see if other conditions might also be included under the manic-depressive or affective-disorder label.

The pronounced role of the abandonment depression in the borderline disorder has tempted some to adopt the theory that this is a genetically-caused, cyclic bipolar disorder, like manic-depressive illness. Stone (111) compared the incidence of depression in the relatives of schizophrenics and manic-depressives with the incidence in the relatives of borderlines. Since the incidence in the relatives of the borderlines was closer to the manic-depressives, it was theorized that the borderline might also be an affective disorder. In my judgment, Stone minimized the possibility that the statistical evidence of depression in the relatives of the borderline would be expected on developmental grounds alone without having to consider genetics.

When Klein (53), who specializes in drug therapy, found that certain antidepressive drugs "worked" on three subcategories of the borderline—the phobic, the "hysterical depressed" and certain acting-out adolescents, he developed the concept that these drugs worked because the disorders were all expressions of an affective disorder with a genetic component.

Much research must be done before any of these hypotheses can be established, but there are certain serious risks to these concepts in the meantime. The borderline patient's extensive use of compliance mechanisms often gives him the appearance of a chameleon; i.e., he changes his colors to match the expectations of the environment. He can all too easily become the tool of anybody who wants to investigate anything. Beyond that, we have ample evidence of early developmental causes in borderline cases that can respond to the psychotherapy, but the work is not simple or easy. The tendency to turn to drugs as an easy way out can be costly, since, although they can alleviate symptoms, they cannot build intrapsychic structure.

On occasion there is no reason to distinguish between the borderline syndrome and the affective disorders, because the patient has both—a genetically-determined manic-depressive disorder and a developmentally-determined borderline syndrome. This type of patient then receives *both* treatments; drugs for the manic-depressive disorder and psychotherapy for the borderline syndrome.

The basic differentiation between the two disorders most often can be made on the basis of the following: In cases with alternating manic and depressed phases, thoughts, feelings, and actions all rise or fall in harmony. Some borderline patients have temporary manic-like states of elation based on the defense or denial. In psychotherapy, the underlying depression they are fighting usually can be identified by the therapist. Finally, one looks for a history of unipolar or bipolar depression in the family.

Differentiation from Psychopathic Personality

The pervasive presence of the acting-out defense pattern in the narcissistic personality disorder and the borderline patient makes it necessary to distinguish their acting-out from other syndromes in which acting-out occurs. These include: organic conditions such as brain damage, psychomotor epilepsy or schizophrenia, where acting-out serves as a defense against psychosis; neurotic character disorder, where it is a defense against impulse, as, for example, with the Don Juan character; and finally and most importantly, psychopathic personality disorder.

A brief vignette illustrates one of the reasons why it is important to identify the psychopathic personality. It will save the therapist a great deal of fruitless labor and heartache. I was a consultant at one of our better medical centers at the presentation of an acting-out adolescent who had been in treatment for six months without improvement. Each staff member reported his/her therapeutic efforts with chagrin and breast-beating as to why the patient had not improved. I observed that he hadn't gotten better because he was not going to get better, that there had been a misdiagnosis; he was a psychopath. The other trap for the therapist in evaluating the psychopath is to become angry at his manipulative behavior and pronounce a critical judgment rather than a diagnosis.

Three aspects of the evaluation of the psychopath will be discussed: 1) clinical factors; 2) intrapsychic and psychodynamic factors; and 3) transference and clinical management.

Clinical Factors

The acting-out of the psychopath, compared to that of the borderline or narcissistic disorders, is more commonly antisocial and usually of long duration. However, it will not seem this way when first presented. The patient himself tends to be unaware of, as well as to deny, his behavior, so that the therapist has to ferret it out for himself. If the patient happens to be an adolescent, the therapist will often find that the father and/or mother are themselves psychopathic but seem to have made a superficial social adaptation in society despite their condition. Not only do the parents provoke, condone, and support the acting-out, but frequently those professionals who should know better also end up colluding with the acting-out. For example, at a consultation at another medical center, an acting-out adolescent whose father was a lawyer was presented. The son stole; the father helped him to hide his stolen goods in the attic. When the boy was apprehended by the police, the father, through his connections with the judge, arranged to have him dismissed without penalty. He was then sent away to a boarding school, which happened to have a psychopath as a headmaster, and he and the headmaster colluded in all forms of acting-out, which ended up in getting the patient hospitalized. There, coming from a prominent and wealthy family, he was treated by the head of the unit, whereas all the other patients in the unit were being treated by residents; finally, this head of the unit bribed the patient to come down and see me for an evaluation interview. This illustrates the extraordinary tentacles that psychopathic acting-out can spread throughout any institutional system.

We used to be taught that psychopaths did not become anxious or depressed, so that if the patient was anxious or depressed, he was probably not psychopathic. This is not so. If a psychopath is in an environmental jam from which he cannot remove himself by manipulation, i.e., he is cornered, he often gets depressed, even making suicidal attempts to manipulate a way out of the trap. The purpose is to get out of the jam or "off the hot seat." For example, a consultation at another hospital involved an older adolescent who was hospitalized as supposedly suicidal because his father had finally thrown him out of the home. The resident suggested long-term psychotherapy; I suggested immediate discharge because the adolescent's manipulative act in getting into the hospital had made the father guilty enough to make other living arrangements for his son, which was the purpose of the acting-out.

Intrapsychic and Psychodynamic Factors

The term "psychopathic personality" is probably an umbrella term, much like that of "schizophrenia," that contains many subcategories of disorder which may vary a good deal in both clinical style and psychodynamics. The etiology at present is considered to be a mixture of congenital, constitutional and developmental influences. A perspective can be gained on two possible psychodynamic types of psychopathic personality from the following clinical experiences.

Fear of Engulfment. A 16-year-old boy was admitted to the adolescent inpatient unit for truancy, temper outbursts, drug abuse and drug dealing over a period of three years. The unit was very efficient at controlling behavior, so that within several weeks the patient's acting-out behavior was controlled. He then became homicidal and suicidal and had to be placed in the quiet room.

An evaluation conference confirmed a diagnosis of psychopathic personality and posed the issue of his disposition. Many were anxious about discharging the patient because of his clinical state. I viewed his homicidal and suicidal state as iatrogenic and recommended immediate discharge. I felt that by controlling his behavior, we had removed his principal defense of acting-out; by having a therapist see him every day, we had forced him to relate to an object. In so doing, we had revived his ancient fears of being engulfed while removing his principal defense, acting-out. Thus he became homicidal and suicidal. This view seemed correct, as he was discharged without incident.

Fear of Abandonment. Another 16-year-old boy was admitted with a suicidal attempt after a three- to four-year history of stealing, drug abuse, truancy, outbursts of temper at home, and conflict with the law. Again, his behavior was controlled relatively soon. His therapist saw him daily, and each interview was filled with projected anger and rage at and vilification of the therapist. As supervisor, it was my task to shore the therapist up so that he could go back and endure the patient's defensive rage.

Over a period of time, one could sense the rage thinning out, and just as the patient began to demonstrate some indirect signs of positive feeling, he eloped; the same situation was repeated two more times: extreme projected rage, which thinned out, the initiation of positive feelings toward the therapist, and elopement. This patient represents another psychodynamic for the psychopathic personality—fear of abandonment. The patient's fear of being abandoned as soon as the relationship began to be established caused him to flee.

In attempting to understand the mechanisms operating in these two clinical types, we can refer to Bowlby's (12) studies of children's response when removed from their mothers in the early separation-individuation stage of development. He describes them as going through three stages: protest and wish for reunion; despair; and finally detachment if the mother was not restored. In other words, after a certain level of deprivation, the child removes all emotional investment in the object and the affect becomes detached from the object. What appears to be relatedness is really

manipulation for narcissistic gratification. In our two clinical examples, what had occurred was that we had taken away the
patient's acting-out defense and overcome his detachment by
jamming in the object. We thereby had revived, in one case, the
fear of engulfment and, in the other, the fear of abandonment.
Psychopaths detach affect from the object in order to deal with
the fear of abandonment or engulfment. Consequently, intrapsychically there is no emotional investment in the object; the
object is empty of affect and is manipulated in order to receive
gratification.

What the therapist then may see as a psychopath's attempt to
relate is really an effort to manipulate the therapist for narcissistic
gratification. Beyond that, the psychopath who cannot experience
the gratification of emotional relatedness turns as a replacement
to various forms of stimulation and excitement for immediate
gratification. Since there is no affective investment of the object,
the psychopath has removed not only from his own psyche, but
also from our therapy, the vehicle and agent essential for its success,
i.e., emotional investment in the object.

The diagnosis of psychopathic personality, then, is usually made
on the basis of antisocial behavior, usually of long duration, without any separation experiences involved, with minimal anxiety and
depression. It can be confirmed in the interview by the therapeutic
technique of confrontation. When the psychopath is confronted
with the denial of the destructiveness of his behavior, rather
than integrate the confrontation and get depressed, he resists and
fights the confrontation, projects, denies, rationalizes and may even
became paranoid and accuse the therapist of attacking him. Sometimes, in more difficult cases, it may be necessary for a short,
therapeutic test to make this distinction between the borderline
and psychopath. It would be well for all of those who do clinical
work in this area to read the follow-up chapter from a book
entitled *Deviant Children Grown Up* (99a), which describes in
graphic and explicit detail the extraordinarily dismal and morbid
long-term histories of those diagnosed as psychopathic personalities.

An argument can be made that there is no difference between

the lower-level narcissistic personality disorder and the psychopath. However, although the acting-out of the middle- and upper-level narcissistic personality disorder may be antisocial, it is more often purely narcissistic or self-centered. The superego of the narcissistic personality disorder functions smoothly, at least on the surface, i.e., he does learn from experience not to do those things which will cause him harm. He doesn't accept that they are wrong if they serve narcissistic objectives, but he recognizes that someone will punish him if he persists. The object relations are present in narcissistic personality disorders, mirroring and idealizing relationships.

The acting-out of the borderline adult is rarely antisocial and usually occurs as a result of interpersonal conflict or as a reaction to separation experiences. The superego of the borderline is punitive, harsh, and often filled with lacunae, but nevertheless present and operative. The borderline patient does learn from experience. The borderline's object relations, though primitive, are definitely present, the patient relating in either a clinging or distancing fashion. The psychopath's capacity for object relations is practically nonexistent.

Differentiation from Psychoneurosis

Although there can sometimes be a problem differentiating the higher-level narcissistic personality disorder and borderline personality disorder from the neurotic, the clinical feel of working with a psychoneurotic is quite different from that of working with a narcissistic personality disorder or borderline patient. The therapist with the neurotic patient feels from the outset that he and the patient are working together, that the patient is an ally in the investigation, rather than an opponent, as with the borderline, or an idol or empty mirror, as with the narcissistic personality disorder. To exaggerate for a moment for purposes of illustration: With a borderline patient, if you happen to make a confrontation which triggers depression, a whole series of possible consequences may ensue, such as the patient's not returning for the next interview, or else returning but not remembering a single thing that happened in the prior interview or denying what happened when it is brought to his attention—in other words, defending against depression stirred up by the confrontation. This gives him the clinical feeling of being an opponent in the investigation.

The narcissistic personality disorder will feel attacked if confronted and respond with devaluation and/or withdrawal; on the other hand, he may spend many hours exhibiting his grandiosity for the therapist's mirroring. However, he is always, at the same time, exquisitely sensitive to the therapist's behavior.

With the neurotic, however, if the therapist happens to make an at best tangential observation when the patient is presenting a problem, the patient returns for the next visit reporting that he had thought a lot about the observation, that it tended to make him feel anxious and depressed, that he went to sleep and had a dream; he then presents the dream and reports more or less what associations occur to him. In other words, he is clearly a partner in the investigation, while the borderline and narcissistic personality disorders, in the beginning, can seem more like opponents.

The intrapsychic structural reason for this difference is that developmentally the psychoneurotic has passed beyond the stage of separation-individuation to the on-the-way-to-object-constancy stage which has brought with it whole self- and object representations and the capacity for object constancy. Repression has supplanted splitting and more integrated and effective defense mechanisms have emerged. The neurotic's principal difficulties spring, then, not from problems in adaptation, as with the borderline, but from intrapsychic conflicts.

There can be, however, some other clinical complications to diagnosis. For example, there may be regressive narcissistic or borderline defenses against oedipal conflict in psychoneurotics who have temporarily regressed to an earlier level. The distinction between them and a borderline patient's defenses can be made by the fact that when one gets through the regressive defenses, what lies beneath them is not abandonment depression and conflict with the mother or father but triadic oedipal conflict.

The next chapter presents a patient with a narcissistic personality disorder whose treatment is presented in Chapters 4 and 5.

3

The Clinical Picture:
Case History and
Intrapsychic Structure

The patient, Frank C., a 47-year-old single professional man, reported that six months previously he had finished two years of gestalt therapy without any definite improvement and that he had always used treatment to fight treatment. He was first treated at age 27, by a psychologist whom he saw once a week for two years. He stopped because: "I didn't respect him." He then saw a psychiatrist whom he liked for seven years twice a week; but he did not change. He reported: "It was all intellectualization; I could talk things away. The responsibility was all mine. If there was any way to get around it, I would."

He added that he felt an inner grayness, an anger, resentment, depression and did not feel good about himself; he felt hopeless about treatment ever working because of his long history. When he stopped seeing the psychiatrist after seven years, he was surprised to note that, despite the fact that he had seen him for such a long time, he missed the psychiatrist very little and had very few thoughts about him or the relationship. He later tried gestalt therapy for two years. He said that he resented the instructions and the various exercises and found himself performing them physically while fighting them emotionally.

He noted that he was absorbed in other people, in things outside himself, and had to have a structure of daily activity as well as a constant supply of friends; otherwise, he would feel empty and angry and depressed. He felt that he let himself down in his general knowledge; he did not know enough about history, politics, etc. He frequently felt alone and helpless and isolated. He was quite aware of the fact that he needed constant "connection with and continuous stroking from other people," without which he would feel small, anxious, insecure, angry and alone; despite this he was aware that he gave very little in these relationships and, therefore, felt isolated and alone. He tended, in his behavior with others in the pursuit of mirroring, to ignore his own wishes, which often left him frustrated. He was extraordinarily sensitive to and intolerant of criticism and, when upset, demanded support from his friends. He reported that he had great difficulty with his office help because he was constantly criticizing them for not providing appropriately for his needs, i.e., his need for perfect mirroring.

He was currently not in a relationship with a woman. He had started dating at a late age, had had a number of relationships with women, the most recent about four years ago, when he saw one woman exclusively. He felt he loved her, but she eventually turned him down. She said she loved him, but felt he was unable to give and unable to love. He said that this left him feeling closed off, empty and unable to respond to her.

He had previously had the identical experience with another woman and, outside of these two experiences, had not had any other close relationships with women; rather, he tended to settle for dating relationships.

He was good at his work and had a number of outside interests in sports, music and art which he pursued, despite the anxiety he always experienced when he had to perform.

PAST HISTORY

Frank was the second of three children from an economically deprived home. His father was described as a loud, boisterous, extraordinarily self-centered traveling salesman who was rarely home. When he was at home, he seemed to be more interested in and responsive to his friends outside the family and tended to ignore and criticize the patient. The mother idealized the father and supported his behavior, saying that since he worked all week he needed to spend his free time with his own friends. She felt the father was always right and that he would brook no interference on the part of anybody else in the family. The patient felt that his father knew everything but was withholding it from him. His father was also very suspicious and mistrustful, frequently talking about how people were "out to get him."

The mother was described as affectively and intellectually dull and empty. She took care of the physical needs of the family but submissively catered to and subordinated the rest of the family's needs to the father's. The patient claimed to have received no emotional or intellectual input from his mother.

He described himself as having been a quiet, obedient, "good boy," who did fairly well in school, rarely ran into conflict with either mother or father, was average in sports, interested in outdoor activities but nevertheless felt: "I was boring; I was missing something; I had a fear of what it would be like 'to be out there.'" He finished high school, attended a local college and then went to professional school, while living at home. He described that "it fit my fear of 'out there.'" Following military service, he established himself in his professional work, where he was both competent and successful.

INTRAPSYCHIC STRUCTURE

Grandiose Self-Omnipotent Object Relations Fused-Unit

This patient's fused unit consisted of an omnipotent fused

object representation that provided perfect wisdom, knowledge, direction and care, a fused self-representation of being without knowledge or ability to cope and an affect of feeling good or special at receiving perfect wisdom, direction and knowledge which was equated with love from the object.

Alliance Between Grandiose Self-Omnipotent Object Relations Fused-Unit and Pathologic Ego

This fused-unit formed an alliance with the pathologic ego's defense mechanisms of avoidance, denial, splitting, mirroring, projection and acting-out that operated as follows: The patient avoided self-assertion, individuation or expression of the exhibitionistic, grandiose self with a defensive posture of inhibition and passivity, looking to the omnipotent object for perfect mirroring. This behavior was motivated by a fantasy that if he remained "hidden," i.e., did not express his grandiose self, which he felt his narcissistic father would experience as a frustration, the omnipotent object would provide the perfect mirroring. While under the sway of this part-unit, his behavior tended to be inhibited, compliant, eager to please, with much subjective anxiety and tension, but also not in touch with his feeling state and operating in the interview mostly by intellectualization. This defensive fused-unit was almost continuously activated.

Aggressive or Empty Fused-Unit

The fused object representation consisted of a fused object that was either withholding or was harsh, critical, attacking and demeaning. The fused self-representation was of being small, devastatingly empty, "a snot-nosed brat," helpless, without capacity to cope. It operated as follows: The patient presented first the continuously activated defensive part-unit. He avoided and inhibited self-activation in the interviews and sat passively, without much awareness of affect, intellectualizing and rationalizing his projection and acting-out of the omnipotent object on me as follows: He could not, i.e., was unable to, activate himself, and it must come from me, as that was my job as his therapist—to provide "the golden thread." This bald and unambivalent statement indicated clearly the totality of his transference acting-out. It was for him a simple issue, and nothing else was relevant.

My failure to provide the wished-for direction and my quiet pursuit of therapy, i.e., either silently listening or questioning him as to one or another of his needs, activated the underlying aggressive, empty part-unit. The object part-representation was projected on me, and I was perceived as either withholding (silence) or attacking and demeaning. The self-representation of being empty, fragmented, "missing a piece," helpless and hopeless, along with his narcissistic disappointment and rage, were expressed by becoming "inert" or, as he put it, "unable to act." We later came to label this behavior his "sit-down strike" attitude. The content of the rage associated with this part-unit was not verbalized with me but was handled by splitting and acting-out on his employees for their "failures to meet his needs." We came to call this his "mission."

When I made observations to further his therapy, he seemed to take them in at the time with enthusiasm, but it later became apparent that no further work was done, as they never reappeared in a later session. Exploration of this apparent paradox revealed that the "act" of my talking was emotionally far more important than the content, for it resonated with his fantasy of perfect mirroring, triggered his defensive fused-unit and made him feel good. Consequently, it was not only unnecessary but even threatening to attempt to integrate *what* I said. In the light of this, it can be easily understood that there was no continuity of theme from interview to interview.

The patient was doggedly transference acting-out his defensive fused-unit. As might be expected, the beginning of every interview was an agony for the patient, because it confronted him with his basic dilemma: My silence left it to him to start; he felt unable to initiate the interview himself; when unable to provoke me into initiating, his aggressive part-unit would be activated; he would then enter the "sit-down strike." On those few occasions when he would try to activate himself, he would shortly collapse with blocking, protestations or ignorance—"I don't know"—and feelings of hopelessness and helplessness, i.e., his efforts at self-activation had activated the aggressive fused-unit.

It is important to note that this patient does not represent the usual or more obvious type of narcissistic personality disorder whose behavior is overtly grandiose and exhibitionistic. These aspects of his personality were "hidden" by defenses and only emerged in bold relief later in treatment as the defenses were worked through.

4

Psychotherapy of the Narcissistic Personality Disorder—The Testing Stage:

"The Sit-down Strike" and "The Mission"

Psychoanalytic psychotherapy of the narcissistic personality disorder resembles that of the borderline in that at the outset, in both disorders, there is no therapeutic alliance, and the therapeutic task is to help the patient convert transference acting-out into therapeutic alliance and transference (see Chapter 9). Although the two disorders resemble each other in that they both manifest transference acting-out, the content of that acting-out differs. The borderline patient acts out in the transference the rewarding and withdrawing object relations part-units (see Chapter 9), while the narcissistic disorder acts out in the transference either the defensive, grandiose, omnipotent self-object fused-unit or the underlying empty, aggressive fused-unit. In the process of converting the transference acting-out to therapeutic alliance and transference, the narcissistic patient passes through the same three stages

56

of psychotherapy as the borderline, i.e., testing, working-through, separation. Further, the three stages have characteristics similar to the borderline: resistance and defense in the testing stage; anger and depression in the working-through stage; and regressive defenses against autonomy in the separation stage.

CONFRONTATION VERSUS INTERPRETATION

Despite these basic similarities, the narcissist's extraordinary vulnerability to narcissistic wounds, his/her intolerance of depression and the continuing activation of his/her defenses dictate important differences. The continuous activation of the grandiose self/omnipotent object defense and the parallel need to avoid, deny or devalue realities that do not resonate with this defense explain why confrontations must be used sparingly and cautiously, as the patient will react to them as an attack which will only further activate defense.

Having to deny the destructiveness of his grandiose behavior to his best interest, the patient will also have to deny the confrontation that brings it to his attention. His ability to perceive his true interest is overridden by the need for defense.

How does the therapist gain entrance to this solipsistic system in order to open it to therapeutic change and influence? How does the therapist help the patient convert transference acting-out to transference, therapeutic alliance, and working-through? The therapist must rely primarily on interpretation of the patient's narcissistic vulnerability as it emerges in the relationship in the interviews. Even so, the patient's exquisite, microscopic sensitivity to real and imagined failures in empathy (or perfect mirroring) on the part of the therapist must be kept constantly in mind; also, when the failures are real as opposed to fantasized, they must be acknowledged.

This extreme sensitivity to the therapist's empathy imparts a quality or texture to the psychotherapy for the therapist that differs markedly from psychotherapy with the borderline. Once a firm therapeutic alliance has been established and working-through has begun with a borderline patient, there are inevitable regressions to transference acting-out under separation anxiety and/or therapeutic pressure. Nevertheless, despite these regressions, an overall feeling or texture of trust in the therapist and the work of therapy dominates the relationship even to the point—on the patient's better days—of his willingness to accord the therapist human errors.

The narcissistic patient, on the other hand, well into the working-through phase, continues to monitor the therapist's empathy, seemingly with a high-powered microscope, and to react with narcissistic defense at the smallest deficiencies. Whatever wisps of trust that had begun to form evaporate in narcissistic rage and disappointment. These responses form the essence of the therapeutic work and give to it a texture quite different from that of the borderline, since the therapist can rarely be sure that his intervention will not induce narcissistic disappointment and rage.

Interpretations of narcissistic vulnerability in the interview bring to the patient's attention his exquisite sense of disappointment at the moment he is feeling it, which tends to minimize defense. Exploration of the repetitive experiences of disappointment then leads to their source: the need for perfect mirroring—the golden thread which defends against the missing piece. Only when a consensus is reached between therapist and patient through repetitive experiences and explorations in the interviews that this need is a projection is it possible to extend the investigation to its ubiquitous presence outside the interviews.

The direction of the inquiry with the narcissistic patient from events in the interview and the therapeutic relationship towards similar experiences outside the relationship is the opposite of the direction of the inquiry with the higher-level borderline, who has a clinging defense. Here the confrontations begin on behavior *outside* the interview which leads to the investigation of the therapeutic relationship.

Having made a distinction between the uses of confrontation and interpretation, I'd now like to qualify by pointing out that it is not a black and white issue but rather one of emphasis. Sometimes one must use confrontation with a narcissistic disorder, particularly where there are many instances of self-destructive acting-out outside the interview. And sometimes one must use relatively early interpretations with the borderline; for example, a lower-level borderline patient with a distancing defense may require an interpretation that the defense is to protect his narcissistic vulnerability. One should keep in mind, however, that using confrontation with the narcissistic disorder and interpretation with the borderline may activate defense rather than therapeutic progress.

The following illustrates in detail how the transference acting-out of the narcissistic personality disorder is converted into transference and therapeutic alliance through the interpretation of the patient's narcissistic vulnerability in the interviews.

The treatment of Frank C., whose history is given in Chapter 3, is presented in two chapters: This first chapter summarizes an account of the patient's resistance during the first two and one-half years of therapy three times a week. It traces the vicissitudes of the patient's defensive, grandiose self/omnipotent object fused-unit as it comes under therapeutic influence.

Chapter 5 focuses on that crucial period where the patient's behavior takes a definitive turn from transference acting-out to working-through, by presenting an interview-by-interview record to demonstrate in microscopic detail how that process unfolds. This account makes abundantly clear the clinical evidence for the components of the patient's intrapsychic structure, i.e., the defensive and aggressive fused-units, as well as their relationship to each other and to the therapist in both transference acting-out and transference modes, as well as some of their historical sources.

THE TESTING PHASE OF TREATMENT

As psychoanalytic psychotherapy began, Frank was quiet, shy and on the surface at least seemed excessively cooperative. He was always on time but seemed to sneak or tiptoe into the office. His initial appearance in general was of being a Mr. Milquetoast, an inhibited person.

The long history of failed treatment suggested that it had consisted mostly of the alternate acting-out in the transference of either side of his object relations fused-units, i.e., the defensive or the aggressive. He either acted out the defensive unit by quiet, subtle, persuasive, and increasing efforts to obtain "connection or stroking" from his therapist or, when this failed, acted out the aggressive, empty object relations fused-unit through being passive and "inert." The acting-out had defeated any therapeutic benefit. His solipsistic system prevailed and excluded the various therapists.

The first objective of treatment was to attempt to make him aware that beneath this need for continuous stroking and connection was an exquisite and antenna-like sensitivity to any and all disappointments of his need for perfect mirroring. It also became clear early on that this seeking of narcissistic mirroring for equilibrium was at the cost of individuation or self-activation, as I shall illustrate.

Soon after the therapeutic contract that I would see him three times a week was set, the need for mirroring of the grandiose self began to emerge. As I expected him to carry the responsibility of reporting his feelings in sessions and did not take over and provide him with "continuous stroking," he fell absolutely silent for long periods of time. When questioned about the silence, he was quite clear that he was mad at me, that I was not doing my job, that it made him furious, and that he was unable to do it on his own.

When I questioned as to why my performing my therapeutic function, which involved listening, upset him so, he said it made him feel that I was withholding, that I was not interested, etc. When I questioned as to where these distortions came from, he was unable to elaborate. When he was not silent, he filled the interviews with intellectualizations almost devoid of affect.

There was no continuity from session to session. When I would make a number of what seemed to me to be worthwhile observations in a given session, the patient would never integrate or respond to them by returning additional material. When I would bring this fact to his attention, he would say that, since what he wanted was a connection or stroking from me, it had to come from me; and since he could not do it on his own, he couldn't see the need to do anything between sessions.

The frustration of his need for mirroring in a session produced narcissistic rage which he would express by what we came to label as a "sit-down strike," i.e., negative silence. He would then return to his office, where he would inappropriately attack his assistants for "not giving him what he needed" or for generally not meeting his needs perfectly. This sometimes extended to his relationships with clients; he would get angry, but with them he would control his anger.

Over a long period of time, a consensus arose between us that the "sit-down strike" in the session was followed by what we labeled "his mission" in his office, to act out with his employees the rage which he felt stimulated by my silence but which he did not dare to express to me. Although I often questioned him about this rage and why he was unable to verbalize it with me, very little progress was made.

Similarly, his need for mirroring caused great confusion of self-representation and object representation in his real life relationships. He had great difficulty setting appropriate limits with his employees and clients and would procrastinate when taken advantage of until he exploded in a narcissistic rage. With his clients he confused personal with professional relationships and had romances with some clients and friendships with others. This behavior frequently got him into difficulties, mostly over finances, when he would also try to continue in a professional relationship.

He elaborated on some of his difficulties during this time. For example, his search for continuous stroking from his friends often led to social activities and interests in which he was not particularly interested. He had great difficulty being alone in his apartment and generally would call a friend to alleviate his loneliness. He felt empty and depressed and often attempted to engage in voyeuristic masturbation to relieve this feeling. Although he was frequently attracted to a woman on the street, he could not activate himself to approach her; the woman had to approach him. Similarly, rather than manage his own financial affairs, he left it to his accountant, who took gross advantage of him. With his clients, he left the payment of the bills up to them and, although he was frequently enraged about lack of payment, he was unable to assert himself to demand it.

For the first two years of treatment, his clinical behavior in interviews consisted of the "sit-down strike" followed by the "mission," with no continuity between sessions and no emergence of historical material. He was transference acting-out with me as he had previously with other therapists, and my efforts seemed doomed to fail. However, when his efforts to get me to resonate with his transference acting-out failed, he turned for the first time from the pursuit of connection and the sit-down strike to trying to activate himself to take responsibility for reporting his thoughts and feelings in the session and to make an effort to understand them.

This movement signaled the giving up of defenses and the re-kindling of separation-individuation. However, as he tried to report his feelings, he became confused, would mumble, start and stop, and eventually say: "I don't know, I don't have the information, the knowledge. I can't do it; the situation is hopeless." There was no way out. At this point he became tearful. His efforts at self-activation had activated the defensive, aggressive fused-unit.

My therapeutic efforts were directed first at making him aware of his extraordinary sensitivity to my every facial expression, the tone of my voice, and the nature of my comments. If I made an observation which did not hit the bull's eye of the target as far as he was concerned, his face would become clouded with disappointment of his need for response on my part, i.e., perfect mirroring. This occurred if I changed my facial expression or even if my eyelids flickered, etc. These minute responses of disappointment then became the focus of my bringing to his attention that his emotional antennae were six miles long, that each had endless numbers of extraordinarily sensitive endings on them and that, for example, should the temperature change one degree or the wind velocity one foot per second, his antenna would pick it up. I began to raise questions as to the sources of this extraordinary sensitivity.

Although he acknowledged the accuracy of my observations and seemed now prepared to work in the sessions, there still was little or no continuity.

This led to his awareness that whenever he had to activate himself and assert himself and give up his need for mirroring from the object, he developed the same feelings of confusion, rage, and depression that he demonstrated in the session in response to my silence.

After about two and one-half years of therapy, a breakthrough finally occurred in the setting of a new and intense romantic interest. He described the woman in terms of physical and emotional perfection and perfect mirroring. She admired him openly and lavishly. There was much intensely satisfying sexual activity. Over a period of several months, as the romantic ardor cooled, she became involved and fell in love with him. At this very juncture, however, he felt that she had lost her perfect qualities and began to find many things wrong with her. His narcissistic glow was gone. He wasn't at all sure what had done it, but he no longer cared for her as he had before. This event made it possible to link his need for perfect mirroring in the sessions to his need for perfect mirroring from the woman. I suggested that what had happened was what happens in the normal course of any relationship, i.e., that as the romantic aura receded, the reality of the other person with her defects came into focus; for him the disappointment these defects evoked dealt a fatal blow to his need for perfect mirroring and led to depression and rage at her, which effectively put an end to his feeling of caring for her. I pointed out that it had more to do with his need for perfect mirroring than it had to do with her. He was angry at her for the same reason he was angry at me—because of the frustration of the need for mirroring. I suggested that no one could possibly gratify this need, and it behooved him to try to understand why he required it.

5

The Beginning of the Working-through Phase:

"The Missing Piece" and "The Golden Thread"

The interviews cover the period of time from the third to the fourth year of treatment three times a week. They will be numbered serially in order to better demonstrate gradual change from transference acting-out to transference and therapeutic alliance, i.e., to working-through. The "missing piece" represents the patient's fragmented self and the "golden thread" his father's acknowledgment and wisdom which he fantasizes will activate his fragmented self.

Interview #1

As the patient's narcissistic defenses were broached, he reported directly in the next interview for the first time the activation of his aggressive, empty object relations fused-unit through a fantasy of smashing a chair in the office: "I wanted you to calm me down and be sympathetic, and you wouldn't and your outrage at my demand would be so great, you would throw me out. You're cold and hard, and in your job as a psychiatrist you have no feeling or concern for me. I demand and want you to care. Your doing your job for me means you are stubborn and no good, dedicated to your own goal, always focusing on your objective and withholding from me. I feel 'give me something; don't just leave me there.' " This expression of feeling was accompanied by tears; however, he could not identify the source of the tears except to say they were a demand. "Hold me. Make me feel better."

He then reported that, frustrated and disappointed with me, he turned to try to soothe his own tensions and to please himself. He decided to take more time off and to get a new musical instrument. However, he still felt this was only a trick to make him feel better, and he envied all his friends who said that their therapists loved them. "I demand that somebody else give to me, because I can't do it myself."

Interview #2

The patient's facing his fragmented self in the preceding interview led to resistance. As he said, "I feel, 'stop the world, I want to get off.' I feel blank. I don't want to be the way I was last week. I won't get from you what I want, and I won't have you condemn me, judge me as being inadequate."

Thus he referred to his feeling that my questions about why he needed perfect mirroring were an attack, and he was not going to open himself to further attack. He then reported having had a dream about chest pain and that he had had an episode of chest pain ten years ago. He thought at the time that he had had a heart attack, but the physical was negative. I suspected that the chest pain was an expression of his feeling that if he gave up the seeking of perfect mirroring, he would die. This pain recurred in the interview as he was expressing more anger at me for attacking him. He again became fearful of having a heart attack. Without exploring the matter, I mentioned to him a prior patient of mine who had had a prominent complaint of chest pain which had turned out to be psychological in origin. For the first time, he reported a new feeling of being more open and accepting of himself, i.e., he was beginning to be able to acknowledge himself.

Interview #3

For the first time the patient started the interview easily and in continuity with the prior session, reporting that in the prior interview he had been like a boil ready to burst. He then began to investigate his need for perfect mirroring as follows: "For me criticism means nobody cares. It means not being acknowledged, alone, helpless, inadequate. It makes me angry, and I want to get back."

He reported, as an example, his anger at his technician who made one mistake with an X-ray after ten faultless years. I linked his need for perfect mirroring from both me and the technician, and his rage when the need was frustrated. I added that even when I asked a question, it seemed to interrupt the mirroring and impel him to feelings of being attacked. I wondered where this came from. I reminded him that he had given no history of being attacked by his mother or father. He responded that he couldn't recall having been attacked, only a fear that he would be criticized for doing something wrong. I wondered why he was so fearful. He reported, describing the fragmented self: "As a kid I saw myself as poor, intellectually, socially and physically."

Interview #4

Continuity was again maintained as he reported his defenses against the fragmented self. He wondered: "Why do I feel like a battered child? What am I hiding from? I'm hiding to conceal my inadequacies. When attacked, I feel I am wrong, not the other person. I am not capable."

I interpreted his need for perfect mirroring, to defend against his narcissistic sensitivity and vulnerability about being attacked. He seemed to have to be perfect or to seek perfect mirroring. If he were perfect he could not be attacked by the object, or the object must mirror him perfectly; otherwise, he felt small, disappointed and inadequate.

Interview #5

He responded to this interpretation again as an attack and re-turned disappointed and angry, criticizing the fee and the treatment. He reported great doubt as to whether he could activate himself, and as to whether the psychotherapy would work, and complained that he felt worse. The depression beneath his narcissistic defenses was beginning to emerge.

Interview #6

The transference acting-out continued: "I talk, but if you make nothing of it, I drop it. It hasn't been validated by you, and I get furious and become inert. I have this incredible vindictive tenacity."

Interview #7

The patient continued his transference acting-out in this session, although his awareness deepened. For example, he began: "I have a resistance to starting this session despite the fact that I know there is a lot going on. I now realize that I express a very vindictive rage at you by not doing it in here when you don't respond to me; I come out with 'I don't know, you have to tell me.' It's the same with women. I see an attractive woman at a disco, but I don't approach her. The same as in the interview, I don't activate myself. . . . Why is it I have to do it [i.e., transference acting-out] "rather than understand it?" [i.e., work through].

Comment: His progress continued in that, although he continued to act out, his reality perception had now improved, and he was quite aware of the transference acting-out. He could perceive its harmfulness to himself and was attempting, with appropriate affect, to investigate why. He was slowly turning from transference acting-out to the beginning of working-through.

Interview #8

The patient investigated further his "hiding defense" against exposing his narcissistic vulnerability and the self-representation of both his defensive unit and the aggressive unit, i.e., the fragmented self. He reported: "After the last interview, I felt more like a peer with you. I felt good, great, but then when I do the work here, that leads to feeling good, and it stops the work. When I left, I could feel the mission starting. Maybe I felt I achieved what I wanted; I've done enough. I don't want to be seen doing something wrong. It reminds me of when I had bedwetting as a kid. I only want to be seen when I'm doing right. Why was I such a clean, compliant kid? In all my activities, ice-skating, sailing, I am extremely cautious. I'm anxious that I will be unable to control myself. I'm afraid my clients will notice if I make a mistake, afraid of being laughed at.

"My father said, 'Why can't you be funny like some of your friends?' I'm afraid of being laughed at for being funny, of being seen screwed-up and in trouble." Now he reported the self-representation of the defensive unit: "Part of me wants to be adored, receive all the attention in the world and perfect affection. Another part [the fragmented self of the aggressive unit] says 'I'm no good.' I have to hide until somebody else authenticates me. I show nothing until I know I'm the best. I love the response. I loved being number 1 in one high school course.

"In my family the style was the opposite: to point out flaws and ignore achievement. To my father and brother, I was nonexistent unless I did something wrong."

This first spontaneous reference to historical material indicates how it emerges, at first in small bits and pieces. The patient now wondered why he was not more involved in the real world. I reinforced the question by suggesting that the way he managed these emotions took him further from the real world.

Interview #9

The patient reported an incident which triggered his aggressive unit. He had asserted himself with a friend, was attacked, and felt small and in a rage at being judged. "I am small; he is big. I am in a rage, and he has my number forever. Nothing I do can change that image in his mind." I felt this report was a metaphorical response to my comment in the last interview regarding his being out of the real world, i.e., that I had attacked him. I felt my comment may have been inappropriate and did not pursue it further at that time.

Interview #10

The patient missed the intervening interview, reporting that he had the flu, which seemed to be justified by a temperature of 102°. He reported his fragmented self: "I've nothing to say. I'm alone, depressed, there's nothing in there, I'll be rejected for whatever I say. No wonder I want someone else to activate me. I'm angry at the way the ticking of your clock disturbs me. I have a cold which gives me thoughts of a heart attack."

Interview #11

The patient reported: "I come here so that you will make me feel good. There's no continuity, because there's no point in thinking between interviews. You're not there to do it for me. I know it's crazy, but I have to do it. What is the purpose of that fantasy? So that I won't be depressed? I have the same demand from you every day. "I don't seem to learn." The patient now emphasized his intolerance of depression. "You're here to keep me from feeling depressed, and I won't have it [i.e., being depressed]. I won't see what you're doing. I prefer to see it as a withholding.

"I know what I'm saying is true and right, but it's also intellectual, not feeling." I suggested that emotionally he was detached from what he was feeling. I then realized that at the moment this comment was wrong, an empathy failure, and I acknowledged it to him. He teared, saying that at the moment he felt better, more connected. He added: "I just realized that my saying I don't know is a direct bid to get you to come in. My father forbade me to say I didn't know and just demanded that I perform. Again, I am with you as I was with him; I think each time, maybe I'll get it today.

"I never faced or face the fact that it can't be there. What would I do with myself then? I'd feel trapped. My mind gets distracted, drifts and wanders. I was a dutiful son; I waited, never asked, hoping that I would get it, but it never came."

Comment: The patient was trapped in that he could no longer continue transference acting-out to relieve his depression but did not want to face the depression and fragmented self either.

Interview #12

The patient now had a continuously activated aggressive unit with the abandonment depression and the fragmented self: "There's nothing going on in me, no motivation, direction, interest or energy. I feel isolated, alone, on the periphery. I give to no one. I have to do it, live my own life, but I don't do it. I had a dream that I was with an old girlfriend, expecting sex. She seemed to go along with me as if I were a friend, and then she said, 'No.' "

He free associated: "No, you can't have that; you want it, but you can't have it. I feel disappointed, resentful, but recognize that she's playing it straight and that I'm the one who's playing a game. What do I want? You to be there, say something, but no, nothing you can say will make me better. Why don't I talk instead of just thinking? To show off, to get a response? I thought about taking a trip, fleeing and escaping, but it wouldn't do any good. I hate it here. My inert self goes in circles, is locked in; I feel helpless; no one cares."

Interview #13

The patient returned to transference acting-out. He again reported a fantasy of smashing my chair, telling me to go to hell and to send him the bill. He said: "You tell me I'm on a sit-down strike, and I'm reporting feelings, and I'm serious." I wondered why the patient thought this when it seemed to me that rather than being on the old sit-down strike, he now was actually working hard to understand it.

The key distinction here was his awareness that the locus of his disappointment and depression was in his head and not in me; i.e., his self-activation had triggered the aggressive unit, and the affect was projected on me. The patient reported: "I couldn't tell the difference." That is, he couldn't tell the difference between transference acting-out and working-through. "I want to be able to follow through on what I want."

I now interpreted that he expected to be attacked for activating himself here in the session and that his activation triggered a fantasy of being attacked, which he projected on me and felt rage at me. "Rage comes from my feeling that you don't care." I interpreted the bind that he felt he was in: He didn't get "it" (acknowledgment) for hiding and inhibiting himself, and when he activated himself, he didn't get acknowledged either but instead felt attacked. The patient reported: "I'm trapped; nothing is worthwhile; it's useless."

Interview #14

The patient continued to monitor the intrapsychic vicissitudes of his fragmented self and his mirroring defense as follows: "I look forward to coming here. Why? There's nothing here. I can't activate myself and there's nobody out there to do it for me. I realize now a woman can't do it for me. I feel my work is terrible. But then, I make plans with somebody, and the bad feeling goes away. I saw a movie where I envied the kid's relationship with the psychiatrist, who was so positive toward him. Again, I feel empty, alone and cannot activate myself."

At this point his depression emerges and he cries; however, it annoys him: "The crying annoys me. It gets me nowhere. It interrupts my train of thought. I'm feeling inert and thinking of dying and aging, etc., etc., hopelessness and helplessness. I want you to say something. I need your voice or I stay locked in the trap. Everything is in your voice, in women, in trips to escape, etc., anything to get away from these feelings; then I feel, 'screw you and everyone.' "

Interview #15

In the last session he described the emptiness of his fragmented self; in this session, he moved into the rage: "Am I helpless?" he asked tearfully. "The tears get in the way." I suggested to him that maybe they were the way, and he replied, "I don't understand. I'm mad at your silence. After the last interview, I was the angriest I've been in years. I wanted to smash things. I'm terribly sad and mad at others. It would give me pleasure to wipe everyone out. I had a fantasy of my dying and you being concerned, and then I felt better; I had another fantasy that you were not concerned, and then I hated you. When I gave my girlfriend up, I gave up someone who cared, and nobody cares. I think I'm giving up the idea of you and others doing it for me, which leaves me feeling hopeless, helpless and in a rage. I push those feelings aside like the tears. When I have to do it myself, I feel thwarted and want to kill and then feel safe that I'm being quiet.

Interview #16

This session began with a dream of my rejecting him, probably for self-activation in the prior interview: "When the interview ended, you were angry at me and walking away. I tagged along. I didn't understand what you said. You turned away in disgust and didn't answer and then got involved with your own people. Then I remembered I hadn't told you I was going to the hospital to have a cyst operated on. I got to the hospital and no doctor; I didn't know what to do. I wandered about the hospital looking for information and then realized that the cyst was really nodes that didn't require operation, and I didn't belong in the hospital, that I had set the whole thing up and maybe didn't need it."

Frank free associated: "The whole feeling in the dream was: I set something up in a vacuum. In the absence of others to activate myself, like in the dream, I'm lost. In the interaction with you, I felt alone, helpless, aware of not being able to manage myself. It was like the time I tried sailing and my hands got very cold and wet, and I couldn't do it and felt helpless until somebody gave me some gloves and showed me how."

At this point I made an interpretation that the sailing metaphor was an expression of his feeling of being trapped in treatment with his self; he felt helpless, miserable, in a vacuum, and interested only in feeling better, not in understanding. Also, he felt that I had led him to believe that was wrong and, therefore, that I had a feeling of disdain toward him for "being wrong." He responded: "Your comments about my being helpless, not maintaining continuity, are taken as attacks. The only way I know you're with me is for your remarks to be perfect. If you're off target, you're not thinking about me, and unless I am perfect, I am wrong." I again questioned why he needed perfection.

Interview #17

He began angry, thinking about crying: "The crying gets in the way, because it puts me in a different kind of light with you. I feel weakened; I think about the bedwetting. I'm mad at you." Tears flowed again. He talked again regarding his fragmented self—no sense of self as an object, no mass to it, no weight. "I get some sense of mass or identity only through others; my mother and father didn't give it to me."

Interview #18

He reported he was blocking his thoughts: "My goal is to be comfortable. I feel inert. This sustains the anger. If I give up the anger, I feel alone, helpless, hopeless, with tears." As he attempted to set limits to the transference acting-out in the session, the tears came forth and he wondered why the tears, as they seemed to have no content. I interpreted that he felt the tears were an interference because they interfered with his mission, i.e., transference acting-out. He asked where the tears came from. I suggested that the tears came from himself, his inner self, which seemed alien to him. The tears increased, and he responded: "The only person I recall loving as a kid was my music teacher. This contrasted with my entire relationships with my family, where I felt so inadequate."

Interview #19

The patient began the session saying: "I thought to make a joke about the room being warm, and I said to myself, 'No, I have to stick to my guns.'" I interpreted that being spontaneous here was self-expression, which interfered with his transference acting-out just as much as the tears did; that in his transference acting-out, he was expressing his mission, his revenge, about not receiving from me, and to be spontaneous and make a joke he would have to give this up; that spontaneity blew his cover that he could not initiate himself, and it also let me off the transference acting-out hook of having to activate him, because he could do it himself.

He responded: "I have to remain hard, cold, aloof and rigid." I then discussed the relevance of this feeling to the beginning of each interview, where he was always posed with the question of whether or not to be spontaneous and self-expressive, or cold and aloof. In other words, should he transference act out or work through.

The patient responded: "If I do activate myself and there is no response or it doesn't work, I'm worse off. I go deeper into my mission, to the feeling of anger and helplessness. He then made a slip, saying he sought perfection when he meant protection; I responded that perfection provided protection, i.e., he did not have to worry about being attacked. After this extensive consideration of his transference acting-out, at the end of the interview, he said: "At work I'm being more realistic than perfectionistic; I don't have to eradicate all the problems. After all, I've been with you for four years, and you're not upset that I'm not better." I pointed out to him that if he felt I could do poorly, then why couldn't he, and he laughed—the first introduction of humor, and the first small sign that the therapy was beginning to take effect and he was beginning to change.

Humor with the narcissistic patient must be used much more carefully and sparingly than with the borderline, since he has such little distance from his narcissistic vulnerability. However, when humor can be used, it can be very effective.

Frank then reported the following dream about treatment: "An old doctor was leaving his office to me. There were no plans in the office, no history; I was absolutely alone, with nobody else there, and I thought, 'Why am I here?' I felt helpless. I thought, 'This has been underway, in the process for a long time without my knowing, totally covert; I don't know why. I'm overwhelmed. An entire office has to be moved in. The aloneness is incredible. Something has to happen, but I can't do it. I must go on, and I don't know why or what happened before. I'm just there, and nothing happens. A goal has to be established. A process has been going on, but I just found out. I set this in motion without involving myself.

When I asked what he thought the dream meant, he replied, "The dream is my fear of what's going to happen. Perfection was my protection." This was followed by another dream which covertly reflected that his hopelessness was diminishing: "I was at a wedding party. There was a wedding party that I should have attended, and I felt guilty about being somewhere else. I was standing in line for ice cream with the girl in front of me. I had an erection. She smiled at me. I should speak but couldn't. We got married and had children. How did this happen? I am not even sure I like it."

Frank associated: "Once I assert myself and make a decision, I have to stay with it. I'm bound to the decision. Better make the perfect choice. Anything else is catastrophe. I have to make sure it doesn't go wrong. Life has to be trouble-free and perfect."

Interview #20

The patient reported further signs of improvement, feeling confident in his self, taking pleasure in activating himself: "I took a music lesson, and it went very well. I was doing it. I was thrilled and excited. At work I felt confident, more involved and relaxed, as I did 'the best I can,' rather than trying to be perfect [shifting from pursuit of the fantasy of perfection to realistic motivation]. As I saw that this came from my work with you, I balked." I asked why. He replied: "It interferes with the mission," and then began to tear. I said: "Like the tears?" He ignored this comment to reiterate that he was feeling much more confident, activating himself realistically at work and that his notion of having to hide was less important, i.e., he was giving up the transference acting-out and beginning to work through.

Interview #21

This acknowledgment of his own self-activation triggered his aggressive fused-unit and the abandonment depression, as he reported in the next session that after the interview he had felt small, alone, and emtpy, and resented having been a good boy all those years, as no one had really cared. I reminded him of his assumption that he must comply with other's expectations perfectly or they would withdraw and recalled that in the last interview, as in a prior session when he activated himself, self-activation had brought on feelings of aloneness and emptiness; in order to defend against these feelings, he gave up self-activation and instead started to comply with expectations that he fantasied I might have. He intellectually referred to his father: "I cherished a single word from him. I place the same premium on your words. They have to be made of gold."

Interview #22

Frank reported more signs of improvement, submitting to the limits of reality his defensive narcissistic self-object fused-unit, rather than acting it out, as follows: He seemed reluctant to start the interview, saying he had trouble recalling what I had said; he then launched into a detailed story of the purchase of a marvelous musical instrument. He felt the salesman was aloof and disparaging, which triggered his aggressive fused-unit and made him feel small and inadequate. Although this might have been his projection, it seemed from his report to reflect the salesman's attitude. But rather than acting out these feelings by withdrawing, he used his reality perception to set limits to the projection of the aggressive fused-unit and turned instead to assert himself and tell the salesman off. Recalling the episode later, he reported he felt extremely strong and then he teared, as he thought about telling the salesman off, and he felt noble, solid, a feeling of freedom from others. "I'm acting on how I feel, not on others."

This was the first evidence the patient reported that he was containing the projection of the omnipotent object on others; this projection required him to be perfect or be wrong, bad, alone and empty and also required him to hide his exhibitionistic self. Instead, he perceived the salesman as a real object and set limits to his disparaging behavior. He began to feel his real self as being assertive and worthwhile.

He then turned again to working-through: "I had a fantasy of you, father and me on a huge stage feeling overwhelmed. I asked, 'What is going on?' I waited for father's approval, and it never came. Mother said father was intelligent. Where the hell was it? All I saw was his hanging around the house in his undershirt. Father put mother down all the time. Mother showed her love for father by never disagreeing with him, even though he was wrong. She lived her life through him. This established her value. Where was she, her personality, her wishes? She negated herself."

Interview #23

I was late starting this session, and the patient saw my previous patient leaving. This frustrated his exclusive mirroring fantasy, and he began the interview with resistance: "You can't switch emotions that fast between patients so that, therefore, you're not with me. I'm not important; if I had started talking, I would have thought that I was talking and you were not there. I get angry and stop."

I suggested that perhaps he was going to do to me what he felt I was doing to him, i.e., if I was not "with him," he would not be "with me." He replied: "When I do put out and get involved . . ." at which point he began to tear and again fought the tears, feeling they interfered. I pointed out to him that he seemed to be fighting the tears. He replied: "Your comment relieved my angry sit-down strike." I then confronted him, saying that in this intense reaction to my other patient he was denying the reality that I don't have to switch emotions so quickly between patients, as my job is not emotional but intellectual. I then suggested that he felt he required perfect responsiveness from me to activate himself, and when he felt he didn't get it, he was disappointed and angry and acted this out in the sit-down strike.

He then reported several efforts to defend against the depression revealed in the previous interview. He had had a date with an old flame, felt momentarily sexually interested in her, but then found that she had another beau and became angry. His anger had led to old memories of her and tears; here he identified for the first time that the tears were related to sadness and loss.

I reminded him of how he had denied that the tears had any content, i.e., depression, and had fought them. The same evening, when his defensive fantasies with the woman did not work out, he had a dream of making love to her in which she said she wanted to be his lover, and he felt big, full, and rich and adored by someone he found adorable.

He associated: "After the dream, I thought: 'Your job is not like that, to make me feel important. I can't do it myself, as I am empty and emotionally debilitated. I want you to take her place, give me that sense of importance and caring. After the last interview, I wanted to ask you, 'Do you like me?' " At this point, the patient was sobbing. "That is always the question: Do you love me perfectly, totally? That's what I need. If it's slightly imperfect, I don't have it, and I feel empty."

He then switched from transference acting-out with me to again begin working through the relationship: "I had to have father's golden wisdom to fill in the missing piece, but there wasn't any."

At the end of this session, I made the mistake of pointing out to him that he seemed to make no distinction between his father, his girlfriend, and me with regard to this need.

Interview #24

He began: "I'm not feeling today. You're not going to feel about me, so I won't about you," referring to my comment regarding my job being intellectual, not emotional. I immediately brought up my comment at the last session, acknowledging that I thought it was a mistake. He replied, referring to his narcissistic projections: "If reality is not the way I want it to be, I'll make it the way I want. I really have to learn to accept reality as it is. I don't like that; it's depressing." He referred to the movie he had seen where the psychiatrist told his patients he liked them: "I want to ask you, 'Do you like me?'" he said with tears. "I know you would say to me, 'Why do you need it?' Accepting the reality of you as my therapist means being left out in the cold. Reality means you don't care and that I do not interest you." The tears were now flowing.

Setting reality limits to his narcissistic projection triggered the aggressive unit with its abandonment depression. Referring to his mother and father, he said, "They didn't have it and didn't give it to me." Again he turned from transference acting-out to working-through. "It made me feel boring, dull and ineffective. No one cares. I want my girlfriend to love me, as in the dream, but she wants somebody else.

"I have the same image of myself that I had as a kid in my family's apartment: can't go out, can't explore on my own, can't see anything happening, nobody cares, lonely, empty, sad." He tried to explore his depression, recalling memories of trips where he felt alone and depressed, but these thoughts led immediately to relationships he had found with people, and the depression disappeared.

I brought this to his attention, outlining his defensive and underlying aggressive, empty fused-units. He responded: "If someone acknowledges me, I feel good, I feel a high, but they have control" [mirroring of defensive, omnipotent, grandiose self defensive fused-unit]. "If someone doesn't, I am low, depressed, empty, start attacking myself and can't activate myself" [abandonment depression of aggressive, empty fused-unit].

Interview #25

Frank began: "After the last interview, I thought, 'Why didn't you tell me that I try to avoid sadness?' I know you must have. As I fantasize myself out of depression, I don't stay with it. I do that rather than try to understand it. I felt I undersood for the first time what the work here is all about. I am supposed to explore the depression. My goal has not been to explore the depression but to feel better by getting approval."

He then reported a dream in which two of his friends were fighting in his apartment, and he just could not get his act together. "I can't get my clothes together; I can't regulate myself." He free associated: "I don't know what I'm doing. I couldn't get my act together. Because my friends were fighting, I couldn't trust them. I could be screwed by them."

He then told of a second incident, in search of the perfect musical instrument, in which he was put down by a salesman, and again, rather than accepting the put-down, he set limits to his projections and asserted himself with the salesman. "Although I told him off, what I felt was 'little me' against all those people better than me. I can't show myself. I can't buy a big expensive musical instrument" [he can't acknowledge the value of his own wishes]. "I don't trust myself, my own judgment. I go to others, no confidence in self-expression without the approval of others." He returned briefly to his father: "I guess I'm still waiting for my father's wisdom. Father is withholding because I don't deserve it. Who am I to be entitled to such an expensive item?"

Interview #26

After the last interview, the patient was irritable and acted out his "mission" at the office, got a migraine headache and then had a dream in which he was at a theater with his classmates. They were bright, attractive, more solid than he had thought at school, and he felt included, good, warm, and accepted; there was no hiding. It was the opposite of how he had felt at school. He associated: "When I go to the musical auction, I want to feel as I did in the dream."

Comment: It seems to me the dream is a response to the session where my comments made him feel included and warm and more self-assertive. He still has no free associations when he wakes up after dreams, and he responds to my asking as an attack: "When you ask my thoughts about the dream, it makes me mad, an expectation I can't meet. Am I conjuring or creating or remembering my father as he was when I was a child?" [at this point he teared] ". . . I'll bet my father complained to my mother about my infantile activity, lack of bladder and bowel control, and all that messy stuff. Even at five I never did anything wrong, but the memory is not available to me. Father was disappointed in me. Mother placated him and negated me.

Interview #27

The patient again expressed his resistance to working-through; in other words, his self-activation produced rage which he projected on me and acted out against by stopping the working-through. He began the session by reporting that he had bought the instrument for a lot of money, felt excited and high, but then became worried that it might not be an authentic antique, i.e., perfect. He then felt that activating himself led to his being screwed.

I suspected that this example was an expression of his fragmented self which had arisen in the last interview, because he had begun to activate himself and work through.

He now reported that when he had left the last interview, he had been angry at me. He had been coming here for four years, and I was still saying the same thing. He complained that I didn't investigate things; that I made general statements that never seemed to be related to what he was talking about and made sweeping statements that made him angry.

I interpreted that he had been disappointed and angry that I didn't acknowledge his efforts to work through the fragmented self, but that actually this self-activation, this working-through, itself frustrated his need for connection and brought on his feelings of anger and disappointment, which he projected on me. In other words, if he was activating himself, he felt angry and alone and could not use me for connection. This seemed to throw some light, as he responded: "At that moment I want your undivided attention so precisely, I feel like I'm going into an abyss and have to have an absolutely perfect thread of gold from you that says, 'It's okay, I'm with you'; if I feel I don't have it, I give up the task."

I pointed out the reality that I was his partner in the therapeutic investigation in order to acknowledge his true self-activation and then I distinguished between the reality of that need and his need for the perfect gold thread, i.e., perfect mirroring. One must acknowledge in some way the true self's efforts at working-through or the patient will give up; at the same time, it must be made clear that this differs substantially from perfect mirroring.

Interview #28

He returned to the next interview reporting that he felt good, that I had shown that I was with him, which was what he wanted, but he was disturbed that the feeling had to come from the outside "as though I won't work unless I have you there. . . . When I was a kid, I wouldn't go to the schoolyard unless a friend was there, and when you say nothing here, whatever goes on in my head ends, and the session seems wasted and I get mad. I work here only so far, unless I feel you're there, just like in the schoolyard. If my friend is not there, I won't go; without him, I feel helpless and alone."

I again interpreted, using the analogy of the schoolyard, that

activating himself and working through in the session was analogous to being alone in the schoolyard, made him feel angry and
helpless, and the flow of associations in his head stopped. I wondered why. He responded: "There is no flow; there has to be an
easier way." He then began to tear and got annoyed at his tears. I
thought the tears indicated he was beginning to take back his
projection and acting-out on me and to contain the affect of depression; however, he still fought allowing himself to feel and experience it. I asked him why he fought it. He replied: "I don't know
what's going on." I wondered how he could expect to know, since
his intention was to fight the feeling. He then spoke of feeling like
being in a dark room without a light, that he had always been a
coward, never had any fights as a kid. On some rare occasions,
when he was particularly sensitive, he had had rage outbursts
if one of his friends fooled around with him. Then he said, "I feel
I'm cooling out; where am I; it came to an end." He had inhibited
his flow of thought.

Then he raised a question about his father: "Did I ever want to
kill him?" He could recall no raging resentment at him. He felt
that it must have been forbidden, because certainly the situation
called for it. He then went on to speak of his brother, who never
paid any attention to him either. He suddenly stopped the working-through and again got angry and acted out. He said: "I've
told you all this before." I pointed out how he had done it again.
He began to investigate the anger at his father, became angry at
having to do it for himself, and turned the anger on me.

Quite clearly, here is an example of his transference acting-out
with me rather than remembering and working-through, vis-à-vis
father and brother, but I didn't make that interpretation. However, he went on to say: "I wanted my brother to single me out
just because I was his brother, but I got nothing. It was like I was
left alone in the schoolyard again, and everybody was pointing at
me saying I got nothing because I deserved it."

Interview #29

The patient's insight deepened in this session. He continued

from the prior session with a metaphor for the feelings of emptiness of the fragmented self that he gets when he tries to activate
himself—feeling helpless, a schmuck, alone, etc. He also recognized the projection of the omnipotent attacking object of the
aggressive fused-unit on the environment, feeling that people were
deriding him. He then reported a defensive dream in which an
uncle who had actually died was portrayed as alive. He had been
close to this uncle. There followed a dream in which he was
carrying his musical instrument without a case and it was exposed,
and he called his brother to pick him up, and then the dream
turned to his being with a lot of his cousins, where he felt involved and very good. He associated: "I felt very good in the
dream, and when I woke up, I felt empty, upset, as if I was
entering a cold world with nobody there. All those connections
were in the dream." In other words, the dream was defense against
the depression brought to the surface by the prior interview.

He then reported two more defenses against the depression: "I
have to fill my time more. However, no matter how much I fill
my time, it doesn't seem to work." Secondly, he pursued connection: "I think I'll call my girlfriend for the weekend. I feel a
longing for someone, but no one seems enough and no activity
seems enough, and I can't do it alone, there is no flow." At this
point he broke into tears, but again attacked the tears with sarcasm,
saying, "Could the tears be the flow?"

He noted that the tears appeared in the session when he found
himself unable to continue activating himself. I now made an
interpretation, starting off with his initial statement that whenever he attempts to activate himself, he runs into this feeling of
emptiness, coldness, is unable to go further and then seeks protection either by connecting with someone else or by filling his
time with activities. As I said this the tearing increased, and he
reported that he teared not only when he couldn't do it, but also
when I talked, i.e., acknowledged him.

He then reported that he was able to stay with the depression in
the interview, although he felt miserable. He had great difficulty
holding on to it between sessions. He continued: "Why should I

hold on to it outside? It's bad enough I have to be miserable here."

This last exchange illustrates a good contrast of therapeutic technique between this narcissistic patient and a borderline patient. If the patient were borderline, I would have immediately confronted the destructiveness to his own objectives of not holding on to the feelings between interviews, but the narcissistic patient would experience this as an attack, and I think he now has enough therapeutic momentum to come to this answer himself.

Interview #30

In this dramatic session the patient moved further into the working-through phase. He began by discussing his search for perfection with the musical instrument, comparing it to his search for perfection in women. He often couldn't make a choice because he felt that there was always someone or something else that would be better.

I pointed out that these two pursuits existed on different levels: one, on the level of reality, where he would like a musical instrument and a girlfriend to enjoy; the other on the level of fantasy, where he looked for perfection which always seemed to lead inevitably to disappointment, whether it was with the instrument, the girl, or his relationship with me.

He responded that the fantasy of perfection gave his life excitement. Without it he felt disappointment and impending death; he didn't want to be left to his own devices. He must either pursue something exciting or attach himself to a woman to feel better. Underneath he always felt he was this dull, worthless kid; exciting women and other sources of perfection gave his self a value.

He then began to investigate the fragmented self, recalling lunch with his friends where they seemed so knowledgeable, and he was nothing and could not activate himself. There was something wrong with him. He didn't know things that he should.

At this point the interview changed dramatically as he shifted spontaneously to his father, "I have to know it all from my father." But, being suspicious, he added, "Am I making this up? I have to deserve what I feel he is withholding from me. He does nothing, but my mother said he was brilliant. I see indirect evidence. He's very funny with his friends, he's a clown, he's performing all the time, he's always on with them but never with me. I have to be perfect to deserve it from him. If I just miss somewhere, if I don't know something, then I goofed, and I have less of a chance to get it. I have to earn it." At this point he noticed that his emotions had started to drift away, and he was tempted to intellectualize. I suggested he was having trouble handling this perception of his father.

He then continued: "If I have to earn it, why didn't I do it? Why didn't I act funny like my friends, as he asked? I behaved like a good kid. I was honest. For example, when my father asked me if I would lie for the family and I said no, he walked away disgusted. He was obviously disappointed with me. It was again as if I had gotten the wrong musical instrument. I said the wrong thing. I should have said I would lie for the family. As a kid, I used to have dreams about concentration camps, and I was the salvation of the family; through my wits I got us out of Germany. But I couldn't do it because I wasn't German; I didn't speak German; I didn't know how; I wasn't smart enough."

He then dramatically burst into tears saying: "My father—I can't be me, being a nice quiet kid. It's not good enough. It's not acceptable, but I can't be anyone else either. I can't get the family out of Germany." Through a flood of tears and anger, he said: "I can't give you what you want." He then reported, after this outburst: "Now I feel strength because I am seeing him saying to me, 'I am sorry I pushed you so far.' I think this is another fantasy to get rid of feeling depressed and angry. It makes me feel better."

I pointed out that the father acknowledged him in his fantasy, and that's probably what made him feel better. I then suggested that perhaps he did not earn acceptance from the father, not because he couldn't, but because by not doing so his negative behavior could perhaps coerce the father into acknowledging him. His immediate reaction to my comment was to inhibit and block, saying that he didn't understand what I was saying, that what I was saying was not wrong but off the mark. I suggested that in his anger and disappointment at my being off the mark, he was retreating and expressing his anger and the disappointment through the "I don't know," to which he retorted: "This is incredible. It's actually happening right here, right now."

Interview #31

The patient reported a dream which had strong oedipal overtones but turned out to be a defense against the disappointment experienced in the last interview. In essence the dream was of being attracted to a woman who was married. The woman finally came on to him and he was passive but finally responded, worried about her husband. She said her husband wouldn't mind, and he appeared and didn't. Later on he was walking in the street; another woman told him how handsome he was; he felt good and got married. This led to a second dream in which he was in his office, with another woman who had recently left her husband, making an impression for his nose which was too large, and he panicked, fearing he might not be able to breathe, at which point he awakened feeling heavy and terrible.

His free association was that the dream was connected to the prior interview, but he couldn't remember what he was thinking about it. He talked at length about his poor memory—was it really poor or was he blocking? He didn't think it was a sexual dream per se. Finally, he recovered the thought that he had lost, that he'd had a pleasant dream that shifted into an unpleasant dream and had ended up being disappointed, whereas the first dream of pleasure was to deal with the disappointment.

He then spontaneously said that he sought perfection because his father demanded it. He recalled again his friend, now a very successful lawyer, bigger than he, better than he, his father's model of being perfect. He was unable to talk with him because he was intimidated by him, just as he was by father. Like father, this friend had all the answers. He had to be careful and good in order not to anger the father. The father wanted him to be funny and rambunctious, but he couldn't do it, it wasn't natural. If he tried to be funny like his friend, he would fail. He couldn't rescue the family from Germany, and if he didn't, he would lose the father completely.

At this point, the patient reported that he was now intellectualizing; he had lost feeling. I pointed out that he had lost the feeling when he perceived that if he tried and failed, he would "lose" father. He went on to say that "trying and failing is like giving him ammunition to reject me, showing my weakness. If I try to show and fail, he erases me." Again the patient cut off feeling. When I pointed this out to him, he said that he had been feeling angry at himself for being so inadequate and stupid, etc. I linked the cutting off with the anger and the perception of the father's erasing him, to which he responded that his father had intimidated him.

Interview #32

The working-through continued as he reported a dream about "needing people to feel right." He then again stopped in mid-sentence and said that he was having a hard time starting; that he was observing himself; that he saw me, the therapist, waiting for him to get to something important, and he felt a responsibility to do it and had to watch himself (a continuation of the transferential relationship described in the previous interview). He said: "I have to be very careful and watch out. If I do anything wrong, you or anyone else points it out and I cave in. It's like being exposed, seen and being called a fool. I'd much rather hide." He then said, "The word 'abandonment' comes to my mind," and reported a dream.

The essence of the dream was that he was searching for some friends whom he missed at a meeting place. They were together, enjoying themselves, not aware that he wanted to be with them, that he couldn't find them, and it was his fault because he planned poorly. He associated: "I felt all alone. It was essential that they be there, and they weren't. They were having a fine time, unaware of me, that I needed them. I thought, 'This is what happens if I don't do it right. It's up to me to do it perfectly to get what I want, because they don't care." And he began to tear.

"I have to do it perfectly to have them close to me, because I care and want to feel connected. It's not essential to them. Even if I do it right, I'm not guaranteed to have a connection. It's really up to their whim; but the only chance I have is to do it right; but even if I'm right on, perfect, it still could blow up. They have themselves together, but they have no sense of aloneness or loneliness."

He now turned to direct images of his family, mother and father sitting in the kitchen talking. He said: "I don't know why I think of that; it almost never happened; we never ate together. They were talking about nothing, saying boring things, complaining about their friends, just plain small talk, nothing interesting, no music, art or literature. I feel scorn for my father's self-centeredness. I'm helpless, know nothing and father's supposed to help and teach me and he doesn't. I want to be noticed and need attention, but that really doesn't matter.

"I recently had a phone conversation with my mother. Her words seemed to have nothing to do with me personally; it's as if she's playing a role as mother. She talked about what a happy-go-lucky child I had been. Who was she talking about? My father was never there. I spent all my evenings watching TV with mother. I don't see father in the house. He was always traveling. Only two times in my life can I recall relating with him—once when he brought some work home and we did it together, and once when he bought me a bike. I enjoyed those two occasions, but that's all.

"I'm left alone with my need; the caretaker can do as he pleases. I felt abandoned by my father, but it seems intellectual. I don't see or sense my mother. Father was bound to his mother and sister, as I was to him; and they abused him as he did me. I see him as much bound to them as turning away from me. He had high blood pressure, and I often thought that I would get high blood pressure; when I notice that my blood pressure is normal, I feel free of being bound to him, which was my reaction when he died —freedom, a release from tyranny.

"When someone else needs me, I feel angry and want to tell them not to bother me, to take away my freedom. For example, when a woman feels a need for me." He paused, "I'm mixing up the participants here—is it a woman? It's as if I'm now in the position of father. They need me and it's my chance to get back, to do to them what was done to me. I'm getting back at him through them."

Interview #33

As the session began, the door remained, inadvertently, slightly ajar; this evoked his sensitivity to being overhead. When he was talking with one person and another could overhear the conversation, his perception produced a whole new third-party system, and he would then try to be perfect for both parties and had to be unusually cautious or the third party would knock him down. He elaborated further his anxiety about exhibiting himself: "It would be noted that I'm not perfect; I would be doing something wrong, i.e., not perfect, and I would be judged and condemned forever."

He then spontaneously reported: "That's why I'm not married. It's the other side of the coin. I would be the judge and trapped with someone I found unsuitable, i.e., not perfect, who would be unsuitable forever. I feel frightened about what people can do to me. I obviously can't defend myself. As a kid I never fought with the other kids."

A condensed narcissistic oedipal fantasy now broke through his narcissistic defenses: "The feeling is like having to confront this bully, the incredible hulk, who attacks me even though I haven't done anything wrong, and I can't do it, but I have to do it. There is some fear I will go out of control and kill him, but that is a thought, not a feeling. Actually, the ambition is to win, kill him, wipe him out and tell them not to mess with me . . . and the fantasy ends with women swooning at my feet, because I have all that power."

However, he then returned to his pursuit of narcissistic gratification. He buys things not for the personal pleasure but rather to show them off to others—his musical instrument, his records, his trips; however, he feels that if he does exhibit himself, he also has to defend himself, to keep his guard up and try to be perfect. In this way, inside he feels that sooner or later he will make a mistake and that it will reveal itself.

Nevertheless, this led to expressions of the fragmented self: "It's like a big empty shell, like an egg—fragile on the outside, empty on the inside—I'm missing a piece; I'm not full except for one time when I got over my anxiety about playing music in front of other people. I played well and felt full. Where does this come from?"

He then began to intellectualize, which I pointed out to him. He returned to feeling by a question about his father. "I saw him as full of all of the goodies. In retrospect, I realize now he was an empty shell, but for me then, he could fill me up—he was my fill." He again started to intellectualize. I pointed it out to him and suggested that maybe it was a way of getting away from his feeling regarding his father. He ended the interview saying that he felt annoyed and frustrated that the matter was so complicated.

Interview #34

This session demonstrated how the patient's analysis of the defensive functions of the grandiose self, in other words his seeking for perfection, exposed that which it was a defense against, i.e., the underlying empty shell of a fragmented self, the disappointment and anger associated with the frustration of this fantasy of the grandiose self. He then projected on the treatment and attacked it. This was probably what was responsible for his moving into working-through for short periods of time but then interrupting the continuity of feeling by becoming intellectual.

He began the interview: "I don't want to do it today. What do I get if I piece it all together? I can't be articulate [activate himself] because my father expects perfection and I'm not . . . only recourse is to be quiet . . . so what . . . so what if I realize father is the core. What happens then?" Here he is expressing literally his disappointment, anger and frustration at the fantasy of the grandiose self. "Why do I have difficulty at being seen?" he asks. "I could only be seen being perfect or I would be dismissed." The bedwetting comes to mind: "I would have to hide it. It is a sign of my imperfection."

He then returned to analysis of the grandiose self: "If my problems are not special and elite and more just like the others, I feel disappointed and close off feelings. My father wanted me to be someone else; I wanted to be me. What's so terrific about being perfect? Staying single keeps me unique and special. A relationship with a woman would put me down, like father did. No one is going to either trap me or dismiss me. No one can get to me, but then I seem to need everyone. If someone would catch me with the bedwetting, I would feel rageful, immobilized and dismissed." He then returned to the fact that if his assistant goofed, he felt this same kind of total rage, that he had failed. He now again felt disappointed and angry and challenged the treatment: "What's going on here? What's the point of all this?"

I thought it was important to do two things here: 1) to acknowledge the emergence of his true self as seen in his efforts to understand himself; and 2) to interpret that these efforts seemed to lead only to the frustration of the grandiose self, depression, and anger, which then led to resistance. He replied: "What upsets me is not what I'm describing but what I want!" I interpreted that the former frustrated the latter, that these existed on two different planes—the former, the grandiose self, in fantasy, and the latter, the true self, in reality—and that the work of the true self-analysis and the treatment—frustrated the latter (his fantasy). He then turned on the treatment and attacked it.

He replied angrily, "Something is supposed to be happening here if I'm doing it right!" I replied: "Something is happening, but it is unpleasant." Frank: "I have no inkling of improvement. I don't want the process—I just want to feel good. If I'm doing it right, where are my rewards?"

Again I interpreted that seemingly the treatment only led to perceptions that he was imperfect, and when he saw this he would become angry and disappointed and stop feeling and begin to intellectualize. Actually there was a process involved. He was investigating how he protected himself from his bad feelings about himself; therefore, the bad feelings emerged as a part of the process of getting to the bottom of the whole problem. He acknowledged that the process seemed to be hanging together better then at any time before in his life—there did seem to be continuity and some kind of overall pattern emerging.

Interview #35

The patient returned to the interview with another ostensible therapeutic breakthrough, reporting that he had a very exciting day after the last session where he felt spontaneous, good, involved, active, feeling his oats as he had never felt before in his life. He seemed to be saying in every way, except directly, that he was feeling good about himself and activating himself without difficulty. I pointed out to him that it seemed to me that he was now able to do it, but was having great difficulty acknowledging it to himself. He first wondered if he was doing it defensively to guard against the bad feelings of the prior session; in other words, was it again based on a grandiose fantasy and connection? Eventually he dismissed this idea. I interpreted that he seemed to be describing what we had come to call his "who me?" syndrome, his difficulty acknowledging and accepting his own self-activation.

He explored further to see whether his sense of well-being was again due to gratification of narcissistic defensive fantasies or realistic self-activation. He said: "There is more to it than asserting myself. I see myself as a reactor. I do it not for myself alone but also to fit in with other people, always conscious that they will be approving it." In other words, whether it is the pursuit of perfection or realistic motivation, its purpose is based on someone else's seeing him and approving of him, rather that on his own worth. "I always see myself through someone else; maybe it's my father." I interpreted the intrapsychic nature of this transaction, that the object was in his head and that he put it out on other people and was either pleasing it or being punished by it. He responded: "Only one or two times in my life could I activate myself to please father, but when I did, it felt terrific, and that was the feeling I had yesterday; i.e., he was now transference acting-out the other side of the coin of the relationship with his father, acting out in fantasy pleasing the father.

Interview #36

The patient reported that the good feeling that he had had in the last session disappeared the next day when he went out for lunch and, attempting to choose a restaurant, realized that he was not able to choose an expensive restaurant. He did not have a big enough self-image. He got angry at himself and wondered why he was not free and then "closed up, became careful, watchful and went into hiding."

He then elaborated that he had great difficulty making discriminating choices. He didn't know how, which made him feel angry and isolated. When I asked if he felt (when he was trying to choose a restaurant) as he did when he was trying to activate himself in the session (trying to draw an analogy between the two), he pointed out that my intervention had again changed the situation. He felt it not just as a question to help him in his investigation; rather, now he was as concerned about me as he was about the investigation. He saw himself and felt himself differently when he was with someone than when he was alone. His self-evaluation shifted, depending on the person he was with.

The unique self-expression involved in having to choose a restaurant or discriminate a personal taste or preference, i.e., this requirement of individuation, triggered his fragmented self, and he felt small, became frightened of "being wrong" and being dismissed and, therefore, could not facilitate the individuative act.

Consequently, he felt angry and went into hiding. In the restaurant, he projected the omnipotent object on the restaurant and its personnel, felt himself as the fragmented self and was too anxious about making an error and being dismissed to enjoy himself. The projection of the aggressive, empty object relations unit from the father on to the restaurant was triggered by the requirement of his self-activation.

He ended: "I'm waiting for you to point these things out to me, but you leave it to me to go further." I asked why I have to ask him to explore. I then interpreted that he was at the same psychological point in the interview as he had been when he had had to choose the restaurant, i.e., he had to activate himself on his own. Here in the interview he tended to wait for me to come in so that he could avoid activating himself.

Interview #37

Continuity was maintained as he explored the fragmented self further. "My feeling is that there is no zest or excitement in my life, no sense that I am and it is all right to be. In a family setting with my cousins, when they talk about things that do not interest me, I feel I know nothing. I have to stay silent; I feel miserable, can't move and am angry with myself. I'm just there, but peripheral." In other words, he was projecting the omnipotent father object on the cousins, and unless he mirrored them, he became the fragmented self.

He then spontaneously went back to his own family setting: "Father was the family, he was this huge center circle, and we were all little circles on the periphery—including mother. Mother gave up but seemed stronger in spite of it. I won't give up and seem weak and cowardly. Father didn't give a shit, and she gave in to him, which made me furious. When I was 16, I heard them having intercourse, heard mother caution father, 'they might hear.' I heard him tell her to forget it, and she did. Her giving in to him enraged me."

I then turned my notepaper over, and he looked up, thinking

the interview was over. He said: "You know, now I see you as the big circle and me as the little circle, and you're forcing me to look up, and I resent it. I have two states—either I am alone, unable to move, feeling I know nothing and can't do anything [i.e., the fragmented self], or I'm following someone else and resenting them for it. Am I still waiting for him to be with me, as I wanted him to be but he never was?" In other words, the patient was still hiding, waiting for the mirroring of the omnipotent object to fulfill his grandiose self. The self-activation, as in the prior interview, frustrated this fantasy, as did social situations, where he did not receive the appropriate mirroring.

Interview #38

He began with his dilemma: "If I do what I want, I'll feel bad, but if I play the game [i.e., do what the object wants], I won't be free, I will still feel sad, alone and isolated." He cited as an example the funeral of his oldest cousin, where he didn't want to go but was afraid that if he didn't go he would feel that they would put him down, and he would feel alone, rejected.

He then reported a separation dream: "I can't get my act together, feel confused, can't cope with circumstances. I don't have information or knowledge." His free association was: "I'm working like a demon to keep myself together but I can't." Although I thought this dream was a response to my forthcoming vacation, i.e., the fragmented self triggered by separation, I made no comment about it. Near the end of the interview, he returned to the issue of separation, saying: "Leave me something for next week or I'll slip . . . here is the substance—I'm doing it again. It was just like with my father—waiting for him to give me the thoughts—I won't recognize that that is not your job." At this point I pointed out to him that he frequently observed that his father had been emotionally unresponsive to him, but he seemed to have no emotional response to that perception, i.e., he denied his disappointment at the father's lack of response. His response to my confrontation was to cut off feeling, to intellectualize, to say that he felt I was putting him down for doing something wrong. I finally realized that he was reacting to my confrontation exactly as I described—he was not accepting it.

* * *

The case presentation is now concluded, as it has served its purpose of demonstrating how the interpretation of narcissistic vulnerability to the therapist in the interviews enabled the patient to convert his transference acting-out to therapeutic alliance and transference, which allowed the working-through process to proceed. Much remained to be done, and there were many further episodes of transference acting-out, but the momentum of working-through had taken over, and the patient was solidly held by the treatment process. As his understanding broadened, his commitment to treatment deepened.

An analogy can be drawn between what is necessary to enable a narcissistic personality disorder to enter psychotherapy and work through his conflicts and the procedures necessary to allow an orbiting space capsule to reenter the earth's atmosphere. The space capsule must be set at the right angle and the right speed at the appropriate time in order for it to leave the orbit and reenter the earth's atmosphere. If any of these procedures are inappropriate, the capsule will not reenter but will "skip off" into outer space. In an analogous fashion, the narcissistic personality disorder requires interpretation of his narcissistic vulnerability in order to give up the self-defeating orbit of his defenses and reenter the world of his childhood to reexperience and work through his conflicts. Inappropriate timing or technique will cause the psychotherapy to fail, and the patient will not reenter the world of childhood but remain locked in his orbit of self-defeating defenses.

6

Narcissistic Psychopathology of the Borderline and the False Self

The prominent role of narcissistic psychopathology in the borderline has been largely overlooked because:

(a) Kohut had no need to stress it, since his theory includes the borderline personality disorder with the narcissistic personality disorder.

(b) Other writers on the borderline stressed that the principal psychopathology was in object relations, to the detriment of the narcissistic side.

(c) In my own work, the narcissistic psychopathology was included in the concept of failure to individuate, a notion too general to do it justice.

I was in the process of reviewing the whole matter while engaged in a follow-up study of treated borderline adolescents (87). Those who improved demonstrated again and again the importance of the narcissistic psychopathology in that their clinical improvement was always related to the gradual emergence and consolidation of the self. Consequently, this chapter first specifies the psychopathology of the self in the borderline and contrasts my own views with those of Winnicott (117) on one aspect of the same psychopathology, which he called the false self.

There is a consensus among clinicians as to the observed phenomena referred to as difficulties with the self—self-regulation, self-esteem and self-expression. Patients report such difficulties quite clearly, and they are not difficult to observe and identify. This consensus at the clinical level gives way to confusion and conflict when it comes to theories about these difficulties: What is the self? What are its functions? What are its constituents and its development? What is the difference between the experiential and the theoretical self? The fact that it is a holistic, overriding concept that goes well beyond such discrete notions as the self-representation of the intrapsychic structure contributes further to the confusion.

We frequently made the clinical observation in our borderline patients of a false self similar to that described by Winnicott (117). However, we viewed it as only one of a broader spectrum of clinical difficulties with individuation or self-expression, difficulties which have also been observed and described by Kohut as defects in the structure of the self (63).

Many borderline patients—adult and adolescent—clearly and concretely express a collection of complaints that are more or less loosely related to self-expression. Some who have these problems cannot complain, as the awareness of the problem is submerged in their pathological behavior. The complaints that are expressed range from an inability to identify their own individuative thoughts, wishes and feelings to all degrees of inhibitions and difficulties in initiating, activating and implementing in reality those thoughts and wishes reflective of individuation that they can identify. There is always an associated defect or inhibition of self-assertion—an inability to support and sustain these interests if, when activated, they come under environmental pressure. There is also always an associated distortion of self-image related to an inability to autonomously regulate self-esteem. It is then a syndrome of the following roughly related complaints:

1) self-image disturbance;
2) difficulty in identifying and expressing in reality one's own individuated thoughts, wishes and feelings and in autonomously regulating self-esteem;
3) difficulty with self-assertion.

Let us pause for a moment and contrast this narcissistic pathology of the borderline with that seen in the narcissistic disorder. The self-image in the borderline is the opposite of the narcissistic disorder, i.e., it is deficient rather than grandiose. The difficulties in self-expression or activation and self-esteem regulation are theoretically similar but clinically different. The narcissistic disorder substitutes grandiose motives for his difficulties with self-activation, and he has much less difficulty with self-assertion. The borderline's difficulties with self-assertion and in realistic motivation are more obvious.

These complaints of the borderline do not exist in a vacuum, although they may sometimes predominate; more often they are presented tangentially by the patient along with his other complaints of depression, difficulty in relationships and functioning, and other symptoms.

The degree of self-image distortion can be used to devise a clinical spectrum from no self-image at the one end through the false self-image in the middle to the poor self-image at the other end.

No self-image refers to those patients whose motivations and behavior were so completely dominated by the need to cling to the object to suppress individuation that few individuative stimuli could break through. Those that did occasioned great anxiety. The patients were quite unaware of this state of affairs until the need for the clinging defense had been sufficiently lessened so that individuation could begin. At this point they would describe themselves as having been "caretakers of the mother" and as "not being a person" or having "no self." An example is a 32-year-old married woman whose complaints were depression, frigidity and anger at her husband. After a year of psychotherapy, as she became aware that she projected the intrapsychic negative image on the husband, she also became aware that she had spent her developmental years as mother's caretaker. "It was my job to keep mother feeling good. She used me as an object for her pleasure. It was as if she or her presence filled the whole house. I had no self, I was not a person in my own right."

The *false-self*, although less serious in degree than the no-self image, still presents difficult clinical problems. It represents a collection of behaviors, thoughts and feelings that are motivated by the need to cling to the object, with avoidance and suppression of individuative stimuli. The patient comes to identify this pattern as his self, and these encrustations can become so complex that it may not be recognized until well into treatment that it is a false self or collection of defensive behaviors rather than an expression of the true individuated self. As a matter of fact, some patients, as they improve in treatment, go through an identity crisis as they begin to lose their false façade and react as if they are losing their true individuated self.

An 18-year-old girl with marked obsessive-compulsive defenses was seen in her senior year of high school for a depression. Her defensive behavior was so well integrated that it took a series of interviews to determine that despite the fact that she was suicidally depressed each night, she managed to carry on during the day at school and at home without anyone noticing her depression. Both parents, who described her as having been the perfect, compliant child throughout childhood, were completely unaware of her distress and were stunned to discover how sick she was. The patient described herself as "split in two"—identifying her daytime compliance as her real self and the nighttime anger and depression as a loathsome stranger she must fight.

A 21-year-old girl, whose long-term depression surfaced at college graduation, presented a façade of the cute, bright, intellectual and intellectualizing little girl who entertained older men with her chatter, while her own feelings were handled by detachment. This role was blatantly acted out with her depressed father, her life task being to maintain his emotional equilibrium through this role. Not until she became aware that she had sacrificed her own individuative wishes, particularly her desire for a real relationship with a man, did she also become aware that what she had thought was her true self was a false self.

A Developmental Object Relations Theory

Developmental object relations theory (74, 76, 83) provides a framework to understand one aspect of the normal development of self-expression and some of the difficulties caused by arrests of that development. The base would be the self-representation which emerges from the fused symbiotic self-object representation of the dual mother/child unit as the child passes through the symbiotic phase (3-18 months), through the stages of separation-individuation (18-36 months), to the stage of being on the way to object constancy (36 months plus). This emergence of the self occurs probably under the influence of: 1) genetic drives, 2) pleasure in the mastery of new functions and 3) mother's appropriate cueing and matching to the child's individuation. As the child becomes a toddler and develops the capacity to separate from the mother, the task of separation-individuation ensues, during which time the child develops an image of himself as separate from the mother. This emerges first as two part-images—a good-self and a bad-self representation—which then coalesce into a whole self-representation, both good and bad. During the rapprochement stage of this process, through the phase of appropriate frustration and disappointment, the child loses the grandiose image of self and the omnipotent image of the object preparatory to moving towards whole-self and whole-object representations. In the course of this evolution towards an autonomous self, the child develops a whole self-image (both good and bad) about which he feels adequate esteem, which is based for the most part on the achievement of the capacity to utilize self-assertion to identify and activate in reality his own individuative thoughts, wishes and feelings.

The difficulties with self-expression in the borderline patient are revealed in psychotherapy as being due to the need to avoid identifying and activating individuated thoughts and wishes, in order to defend against the abandonment depression that such activation would trigger. This sacrifice of self-expression to defense adds an additional negative increment to the already negative self part-image of the borderline patient as a result of the operation of the withdrawing object relations part-unit (WORU), i.e., no approval but rather "punishment" from the mother for signs of self-expression.

To compensate for the fact that self-expression is not available for motivation, the patient turns instead to the alliance of rewarding object relations part-unit (RORU) and pathological ego which, while providing him with a defense against the abandonment depression, at the same time provides him with responses to deal with the environment—a form of adaptation. As these patterns become familiar, stereotyped and repetitive, the patient identifies them as his self. But it is a false self based on a need for a form of adaptation that provides a defense against individuation, rather than one which is an expression of the solutions arrived at by the dynamic experiment and interplay between the evolving individuating self and the environment.

Our follow-up reports of successfully treated patients demonstrated that, as the rage and depression are worked through, the patient begins to separate and individuate, and the self gradually emerges and assumes its functions. The patient develops new thoughts, wishes and feelings (individuation or self-expression), identifies them and assertively activates them in reality, thereby turning away from his old rewarding unit/pathological ego alliance to use his new behavior. Over the course of time there is eventual consolidation of the self. We were able to observe and describe the gradual emergence and various degrees of consolidation of the self which paralleled the patient's clinical improvement.

Let us now turn to Winnicott's view of the false self. Winnicott described a clinical state of the false self as follows: A patient, although quite successful in external adaptations, had the feeling that she had not started to exist, that she had always been looking for a means of getting to what she called her true self. Winnicott emphasized that the link between intellectualizing and the false self created a special danger—a deceptive clinical picture in which there is seemingly extreme external success so that it is difficult to impossible to believe the real distress of the person concerned who feels "phony, the more phony the more successful he is." He dramatized the point by reporting a patient who had much futile analysis on the basis of the false self, cooperating vigorously with the analyst who thought this was the whole self. The patient said, "The only time I felt hope was when you told me that you could see no hope, and you continued with the analysis." He emphasized that in psychoanalysis it is possible to see analyses going on indefinitely because they are done on the basis of work with a false self.

Winnicott's theory of true and false self relied on Freud's division of the self into a part that is central and powered by the instincts, the true self, and a part that is turned outward and related to the world, presumably the false self. This definition springs from structural theory and poses a false dichotomy. The true self emerges as an entity, reflecting the individuation process and probably involves part of the outside world that is internalized alongside of the instincts.

In his development of the concept of the true self, however, Winnicott seems closer to the point. For example: "The true self is the theoretical position from which comes the spontaneous gesture and personal idea. The spontaneous gesture is the true self in action. Only the true self can be creative and feel real."

This concept of the true self goes awry, however, in his description of what he calls the normal equivalent of the false self: "There is a compliant aspect to the true self and healthy living, an ability of the infant to comply and not to be exposed, an ability to compromise. . . . The equivalent of the false self in normal development is that which can develop in the child into a social manner, something that is adaptive" (117). This analogy is an error because in normal development the true self, the separated individuated self, has a sense of being alert, alive, creative, spontaneous and real and through its ego functions interacts with the environment and does form adaptations and compliances. The true self can comply or adapt without necessarily compromising its essence or integrity.

Winnicott felt that the defensive function of the false self was to hide and protect the true self. I do not feel that this is so because there is not at this point any true self. The true self is in a state of limbo or atrophy—it is only a potential. The defensive function of the false self is to rationalize and provide a false sense of identity for those regressive, compulsive behaviors that reflect the adaptive side of the RORU/pathological ego alliance necessary to defend against the abandonment depression.

In his discussion of etiology, Winnicott described the crucial variable: "The good enough mother meets the omnipotence of the infant and responds to it. A true self begins to have life through the strength given to the infant's ego by the mother's implementation of the infant's omnipotent expressions" (117). In more current idiom, the true self begins to have life through the mother's provision of reward and approval for steps toward separation-individuation. This spurs individuation and gives a sense of a true self as the infant begins to separate from the mother.

Winnicott states:

> The mother who is not good enough is not able to implement the infant's omnipotence and so she repeatedly fails to meet the infant gesture, substituting her own which is to be given sense by the compliance of the infant. This compliance on the part of the infant is the earliest stage of the false self and belongs to the mother's inability to sense her infant's needs (117).

Again, in more current idiom, the mother's withdrawal of approval for separation-individuation produces an abandonment depression. However, since the mother rewards regressive clinging, the child defends himself against the depression by regressive compliance with the mother's projections, thus setting up a system of regressive, pathologic defense mechanisms—avoidance, denial, clinging, acting-out, splitting, projection.

The image of the rewarding mother is internalized as one part of a split object relations unit—the rewarding unit—which allies with the regressive defense mechanisms to form a defense against the other part of the split object relations—the withdrawing unit. This alliance, which defends against depression, becomes the basis for the false self. Neither of the part-self images of the two units is the true self since the latter, a developmental achievement, only comes about through separation of the self-image from the maternal image, based on growth and development through the mode of self-assertion, facilitated by the mother's mirroring and matching responses. The child develops a false self not to hide the true self, since the true self has not emerged, but to rationalize the adaptive function of his regressive defenses against the abandonment depression—a depression created by his efforts to develop a true self in the first place. This false self reacts to the mother's projections with compliance, developing a parallel and complementary set of pathologic defense mechanisms. This intrapsychic system is then internalized and projected on the environment and constantly reactivated so that the infant may develop a false self which does relate to external reality on the same basis as the infant's false self related to the mother.

Winnicott pointed out that in extreme examples there is no spontaneity but mainly compliance and imitation; there is concreteness with little use of imagination and symbol formation. As he illustrated, there can be varying degrees of the false self and, sometimes, as in the as-if personality, the false self can be mistaken for the whole personality. In other cases, for example with actors, there may be a kind of sublimation. He stressed that the true self had the capacities of spontaneity, creativity and the use of symbols.

Certainly creativity and spontaneity spring from full individuation, where the self-assertion is unfettered and free to apply itself.

Let us now answer the six questions that Winnicott raised about the true and false self.

1) *How does the false self arise?* The mother's libidinal unavailability for the child's efforts toward separation-individuation during that crucial phase of development produces the abandonment depression, against which the child defends by conforming to the mother's projections, which enable her to continue to cling—through projecting, splitting, acting-out, denial and avoidance. These regressive pathologic mechanisms enabling the mother to continue to cling produce a developmental arrest, but they also relieve abandonment depression and separation anxiety and enable the child to "feel good," as if he were receiving supplies. These defense mechanisms—the alliance between the rewarding unit and the pathologic ego—become rationalized as the child's self, but it is a false self.

2) *What is the function of the false self?* As described above, its function is to defend against separation anxiety and abandonment depression.

3) *Why is the false self exaggerated or emphasized in some cases?* It will be exaggerated depending upon the exaggerated projections of the mother or perhaps some combination of constitutional inadequacies of the child and exaggerated projections of the mother.

4) *Why do some people not develop a false self system?* If there are no constitutional inadequacies and the mother provides adequate mirroring and approval for separation-individuation, there will be no need for a false self system.

5) *What are the equivalents to the false self in normal people?* There are none.

6) *What is there that could be named a true self?* A self-representation that is whole, both good and bad and based on reality, that is creative, spontaneous and functioning through

the mode of self-assertion to regulate self-esteem in an autonomous fashion.

THE INTERNALIZED SPLIT OBJECT RELATIONS PART-UNITS OF THE FALSE SELF

Patients with a false self have an intrapsychic structure that consists of rewarding and withdrawing object relations part-units which may, though they vary in their content, present a more or less characteristic presentation as they emerge in transference acting-out. Initially one sees the rewarding object relations part-unit projected on to the therapist with a clinging transference which may be gross and obvious or much more subtle. When confrontation sets limits to the rewarding object relations part-unit projection or the clinging transference, what quickly emerges in projected form is the withdrawing object relations part-unit. The origins and development of the clinical false-self image as it relates to the two part-units then become clear as they are recapitulated in the transference, as illustrated below.

CASE ILLUSTRATIONS

Susan D.

Susan D., a 35-year-old woman who had had three years of analysis and two years of psychotherapy, complained of depression, difficulty in being alone and managing on her own, a need to be dependent on others and difficulty in close relationship with men. Her mother had been psychotic and was hospitalized several times during the patient's early childhood; her father was a school principal.

The patient's first transference-acted-out behavior was to project the rewarding unit (RORU) on me, presenting her false self, to behave as an intellectualized little girl who was eager to please and comply. There was, however, little or no genuine affect. She tried to manipulate me to give her advice and directions and to provide various kinds of special exceptions for her. My confrontation of her need for these special activities immediately triggered the withdrawing part-unit, which was punitive, critical and rigid almost to the point of being paranoid.

She expressed the negative object representation of the withdrawing object relations part-unit (WORU) by accusing me of being extremely critical of her, of putting her down, and the negative self-representation by accusing me of not being interested in her, of considering her boring, not worthwhile listening to, etc. The issue of manipulation came to a head when she requested a postponement of payment of her bill, as her father had not yet given her the money. I pointed out that the arrangement was between her and her father and not between myself and her father and, therefore, that I would expect her to pay on time; she should deal with her problems with her father; she was asking me to take over her responsibility.

This confrontation led to a furious outburst of anger at my being greedy, rigid, uncaring, etc.; she claimed that all of her friends were in treatment, and many of them owed their therapists three or four months' worth of bills. By the end of the session, however, as her rage subsided, when I questioned the reason for such anger and disappointment, she verbalized her wish to be special to me, which led to the history of similar maneuvers with her father in order to be special to him.

She freely admitted that this behavior was not spontaneous and self-expressive but was put on to get the desired response, that what she really felt about herself was that she was bad, ugly, disgusting, of no interest, underneath which lay feelings of hopelessness and helplessness.

At the same time, I pointed out that whenever she expressed a spontaneous thought or feeling in a session (her true self), she would immediately either assume I was critical towards it (projection of WORU), or she would adopt the most punitive, critical attitude possible towards her own thoughts and feelings. As she became aware that this negative, punitive attitude (WORU) existed in her head and that she was defending against it by projecting it on me and that the clinging was a defense against the projection, the self-image of the withdrawing unit emerged further, and her feelings were that her self was dull, vapid, empty.

I anticipated that, her projection and acting-out having been controlled, she might now begin to remember and review some of the past history of this negative self-image with mother and father. Instead she presented a dream of rats lodging in her hair which frightened her and which she wanted to be rid of. Her associations led to the idea that the rat's nest was those early relationships with the mother and father which she had attempted to avoid by acting-out.

Without affective contact with her memory, she remembered quite clearly that her father had been punitive and critical and her mother flat and affectless. She had spent a lot of time with her mother and had felt that she had to stimulate her mother in order to keep her from withdrawing. At the same time, her mother would infantilize her by letting her stay home from school and by not insisting that she take care of her room, etc.

Part of the compact between the psychotic mother and the child was that the patient suspend her own reality perception in order to take on the mother's psychotic perceptions of reality, reinforcing the symbiotic bind. This was reflected in treatment a number of times, where the patient insisted that whatever she felt was true objective reality; objective reality did not exist in its own right.

In one of these discussions, for example, she had asked for another position at her job. Her supervisor felt that she was not yet qualified and refused to make the change for her. She was convinced that he did it because "he was out to get her." I suggested some other possibilities, such as that she might, in fact, not be qualified. She began to integrate this confrontation and then reported in the next session a dream: If she went along in any way with the discussion, she would be attacked by the devil.

As her intellectualized defenses were confronted, the projection of the withdrawing unit on the therapist became more consistent and more intense. The intellectualizations and the manipulations to be special disappeared, but the patient began to feel more depressed and angry: "You do not encourage feeling here. I have no emotion; I can't do it myself; I feel I'm in a vacuum, that all the air has been sucked out."

She would then have violent fantasies of destroying me, wanting to have a temper tantrum but not being able to, questioning why she had to do the treatment herself, saying that I was cold and uncaring and asking too much, even cruel and sadistic, and that she would like to hurt me as I was hurting her.

Her distorted perception that feeling was tantamount to objective reality was a defense against engulfment by the mother and then by the therapist, as well as reinforcement of the symbiotic compact with the mother to suspend her own reality perception in order to reinforce the symbiotic bind. As these defenses were confronted and the withdrawing unit of the self-image began to emerge, her statement that she could not do it herself was a projection onto therapy from the original interaction. The mother's libidinal unavailability made it impossible for her to individuate, which was then reinforced by the extremely negative images taken first from the mother and then condensed and combined with the critical father, i.e., to forego self-expression in the service of complete incorporation of the mother's projections as her internalized object.

As the withdrawing part-unit began to emerge, she expressed its self-images in metaphors: a kitten hit by a baseball bat; a piece of feces; unable to give to herself; willing to throw herself away in order to feel better. One might anticipate that this emergence of the withdrawing unit in the interviews would lead to working-through.

However, the acting-out defenses of the false-self patient are extraordinarily tenacious. As the frequency of interviews increased from two to three times a week, thereby increasing the therapeutic pressure on her defenses, the patient increased her resistance. She acted out by "throwing herself" into "instant intimacy" with a man. She met and slept with him the weekend before starting three times a week. She reported that he was a nice person who, however, was opposed to psychotherapy. She added that she was afraid I would attack her relationship with him as antitherapeutic.

It seemed that the prospect of containing and feeling the withdrawing unit in her head had activated her defenses of splitting and acting-out. The boyfriend became the good object which she feared losing, and the treatment became the bad object which she was afraid of facing. She had managed to externalize the conflict, and there was nothing internal to analyze.

It quickly became clear that she was allowing this boyfriend to run the relationship and doing very little to support her own self-interest, despite her efforts to conceal this fact. The defensive effectiveness of her acting-out is seen in the fact that the content, i.e., the withdrawing part-unit/negative self-image had disappeared from the sessions. I took no position on the boyfriend but instead tried to investigate her wish for me to attack it, with little success.

Finally, after a period of eight weeks, when she slowly began to reveal the degree to which she had allowed her self-interests to wither in the relationship, I began to point out how destructive this was to her. She again accused me of attacking the relationship and then had the following dream: "I was feeding a cat with a fish hook but acting like I'm doing something else." Her free association to this was: "The pain of breaking up the relationship is like tearing the hook out."

I now interpreted the defensive function of her acting-out: She had set up the relationship to defend and get rid of the bad self-image rather than face and talk about it in sessions. She responded angrily, saying I was intruding and coercing her to do something. I pointed out that she was turning on me in anger to avoid facing what I was telling her regarding herself. She began to cry and said that she felt helpless about the bad feelings about herself, didn't know what to do about them, was afraid she could drown in them. They took over. She was afraid she might go crazy. Her self-image was that of an undesirable insect. She could be that way by herself, but in a relationship she had to push herself around. She had had so much disappointment in relationships that she didn't want to take a chance again.

She then elaborated that to look at the bad feelings would be to do something very frightening, that she wanted to be sure "someone would be there." I asked her why, and she said she was afraid.

She recalled fears at age five of burglars in the basement, dreams of being overpowered and hurt and helpless and being chased by gorillas and visions of dogs attacking her. She couldn't tolerate the bad feelings about herself; her whole identity was a protection against them. She had walled off part of herself to deal with those fears and breaking open that wall threatened her identity.

This led to a dream of "watching children" at the edge of the waves and being worried about them being overtaken and then seeing that they were doing okay.

She freely associated: "I feel less defensive and paranoid and frightened with you today. I used to have dreams of being over-whelmed by waves. The bad feelings seem less frightening or I am beginning to re-own them." She reported a fantasy of my attacking her and strangling her if she did not agree with my criticism of her.

In the very next interview she came in attacking herself, and I pointed out that the newfound comfort she had developed in the prior session led to her attacking herself, that either she attacks herself or expects it from me. She replied: "If I don't do it, it will come from nowhere as a surprise, to hurt me." She then reported a dream of floating down a river in a raft, being relaxed with herself when Indians appeared from behind some bushes and killed her.

She associated that she had a sense of the world being malevolent and if her reports to me didn't fit together perfectly, it would leave an opening so I could attack her. She treated herself as an object, had cut off all feelings about it and become a computer; she cuffed herself around like the kitten with a bat. This discharge in the session led to an emergence of her true self, as she suddenly said: "Suddenly I feel so good; I want to jump up and do what I want to do, and I feel for the first time gratitude to you for getting me this far. She then returned to work on the bad feelings about herself as being slow, boring, a mole, etc., and it became possible to show how she was throwing herself away with the boyfriend as she was attacking herself in the sessions. When she heard of a psychiatrist's suicide in the newspaper, she became anxious about my mental health: Would I commit suicide if she went into this abyss about the bad self? Would I be there to help her out?

She visited her mother which stimulated some additional history: that her mother was without affect, was always sloppy; that when she was a child her mother had her do all the cooking, sewing and cleaning up at home; that her brother was a homosexual. Her mother failed to support her in her wish to continue her education. When I expressed surprise, as parents are generally positive about their offspring continuing their education, she became extremely depressed and said that different parents had different values, which I challenged, saying it's not a matter of values. This led to her need to protect her mother: "One part of my mother is a witch; she put out a view of herself and the world which was very particular, and she required that I join her." Then she said she didn't know how and it's not allowed to figure her mother out; it was too close to her and too big.

She reported an old, repetitive dream: At age five a witch was at the door—"I was scared that the witch would see me." This led to a fantasy of a gang of boys in her yard attacking her and beating her up. As she tried to investigate the relationship with the mother, she felt more and more depressed and helpless. She recalled that the mother was intrusive, giving her no privacy; that mother was both detached and overprotective at the same time; that she'd had fantasies of hating her mother since the prior interview: "I was an object to mother; there was no respect for myself. When mother made father the villian, to disagree with mother was to be a bad person." She reported a fantasy of wishing she were blinded so she wouldn't see these painful perceptions: "I don't know what's reality anymore; I feel like I'm starting to lose my mother; I see her as bad, different from ever before. The positive image of her is being undermined. I'm challenging my perceptions of what mother did when I was growing up."

How the patient turned reality inside out to defend against her perceptions of the mother was indicated by the following dream: "You, me, my father and mother are in a hotel. You took off your shirt and wore panty hose to stimulate me sexually. My father said, 'That's crazy, he's going to have a breakdown,' and you did. I said to my father 'but he helps me a lot.' "

Her free association was: "It would be a relief for me if you were a phony and what you said wasn't so. I wouldn't have to deal with you. I'd have fewer conflicts. I feel panicky and backed against the wall here, frightened of seeing certain things and losing my flexibility. I'm not safe, I will be attacked."

She then reported a revealing incident where she found herself unable to stand up to an angry, paranoid attacking colleague and then found herself taking on this colleague's point of view— probably as she did with the mother: "I didn't want to stand separately and confront her, so I took on her point of view. I'm frightened to use my own perceptions. You keep coming closer and closer here to something that frightens me. I had a fantasy that if I start seeing and expressing things, if I genuinely see them, someone will kill me."

She then defended against this anxiety by going back to talking about the boyfriend, how he was all good and I was hostile to him and wanted to attack him. I interpreted that she seemed to want to throw herself away both with the boyfriend and in treatment and yet still fulfill herself. I pointed out that this was impossible. I suggested that the throwing away was a defense against the anxiety expressed in the last session related to her true perceptions of her mother, and she had to stop throwing herself away in order to face and work through the separation anxiety. She responded: "It's hard to imagine my not selling myself and getting what I want."

She responded in the next interview in further defense, on the subject of being able to throw herself away with the boyfriend: "Why can't you be more flexible?" I pointed out that there can be no flexibility in the perception that not supporting herself is harmful. She responded that she was too frightened if she asserted herself, that he would not want her, nobody would want her. I wondered why she felt she did not have a right both to feel what she wanted and to do what she wanted.

She reported in the next session feeling that my comments about her rights made her feel that the treatment was more her own, that she didn't have to comply or be judged. Then she went on, however: "It's a fact of life that I'm an insect, and I have to work around it; that's the way I am. What is there to understand or change? I see the way I am. How come you don't?" It finally emerged that she felt I was telling her to end the relationship because I was saying she must support herself, which to her was tantamount to ending the relationship. I pointed out how her fear of abandonment caused her to turn her reality perception around.

The next few interviews, without going further into the withdrawing unit, she reported greater confidence in herself, better ability to take care of herself, being more real, not throwing herself away so much. This led to her expression of anxiety in the transference: "I'm frightened of believing that what you say is real and being disappointed. I've been conned before; the other person is laughing at me for being gullible, and how much I care. Mother laughs at my caring, how cute it was. I hate to let somebody see I care. I feel exposed and caught, with my pants down."

These changes might suggest that the patient would now proceed more directly into the working-through phase. However, this is exactly what does *not* happen with the false self patient. There remained much more resistance that had to be worked through.

To summarize, the patient's false self contained a superficial appearance of relatedness which was based on the following split in the internalized object relations unit: First, there was a rewarding unit with an object representation derived from a psychotic mother who had responded to stimuli from the child with infantilizing behavior, the self-representation of being a special child who is indulged and loved, linked by the affect of feeling special. This was then condensed with a similar response on the part of the father who infantilized the daughter. The withdrawing object relations unit contained the other side of the relationship with the mother: a maternal part-object representation who withdrew unless the patient stimulated her, combined with the father who was critical and a self-representation of being uninteresting, unworthy, alone, with an affect of rage and depression. When the intellectualized false-self behavior (motivated by the rewarding part-unit) is confronted in treatment, it automatically led to the projection of the underlying withdrawing object relations part-unit.

Michael E.

A second example concerns Michael E., a 50-year-old writer with a depression. He had had two periods of analysis based on a false self, the first in his twenties for four years and the second in his thirties for nine yearss. The clinical false self of this patient was extremely subtle, complicated, and difficult to identify, since he had had treatment in addition to the 13 years of analysis mentioned above and had written a lot on psychiatric disorders. He could present an excellent and convincing intellectual façade. Over a period of time, it became clear that he was projecting an omnipotent rewarding part-unit on me. He overreacted to most of my comments, keeping his anger and his depression out of the sessions.

The clinical picture started to be clarified through his discussions of conflicts with his wife, whose hostile, inappropriate criticism he tolerated without objection. When I asked why he didn't object to her behavior, it turned out that in certain respects she was expressing how he felt about himself, i.e., guilty, inadequate, incompetent, and no good.

Investigation of this led back to his mother, who had had severe birth trauma when he was born and had blamed him for her inability to have more children. This reinforced early separation-individuation problems by inducing feelings of guilt and inadequacy about himself which he could relieve only by fulfilling the mother's expectations that he make up for her feelings of inadequacy by "taking care of her" and by being very successful. His father, with a severe narcissistic disorder, paid little attention to him. His rewarding unit was a massive projection of maternal expectations with massive compliance, producing severe inhibition of individuation.

The completely negative and hostile attacking attitude of his withdrawing object relations part-unit to separation-individuation or self-expression emerged in the following manner: I had had a discussion with him of some writing he had begun as a new experience of activating himself in his profession, and he mentioned that I seemed to have a positive attitude towards what he was able to do, which helped him cope with his own negative self-image. He then had a dream in which he was in a strange city—he felt free; he could be on his own, set his own hours, be unhurried and unpressured. His associations: "It's the opposite of my pressured life. It's the ability to be free and on my own, but I feel that free time is bad news and will get me into trouble.

"This whole idea of self-expression, being free, it's like opening the gates of a prison. I feel I'm afraid I'll go out of control. It's succumbing to my own wishes." The patient's extensive identification with the withdrawing object relations unit had impelled him to see his own separation-individuation wishes as evil, bad, wrong.

He continued to talk about how to him fun was danger, that he was both jailer and prisoner, that he kept himself under tight control because letting go brought out such enormous anxiety.

He then used the analogy that he was a toiler or laborer in life. He did what was expected. The other option was to be wild, out of control. I questioned: What about the man who has all these potentials but hones them and disciplines them in a sublimated way?

He reported that many of the so-called choices he had made in his life were not free choices at all but were the result of what was expected, that underneath he resented the work of college and graduate school and that, once he got into the profession, he again did what was expected to "get ahead," rather than what he wanted to do.

A consequence of this form of adaptation—avoidance of individuation—was that his life was not providing the gratification and pleasure he had hoped it would. He blamed this on "the way life was" rather than on his own avoidance of individuation.

The patient began to investigate his avoidance of individuation at work with a rationalization: He viewed work as being "plodding, pedestrian, hard and boring." I confronted that he was denying the pleasure involved in work. He returned the next session, furious at me for "being realistic and forcing him to work." He had to work harder in order to pay me; i.e., I have it easy and he has it tough. He then reported being disappointed that I hadn't protected him and said resignedly that there was no magic. I pointed out that he was devaluing me in order to avoid looking at the frustration of his own wishes. I was either over-protecting him or attacking him; there didn't seem to be any in-between.

He following through in the next session to detail his avoidance at work, his difficulty in pursuing a line of thought and in keeping himself to the task. He felt unable to write, to choose, to commit himself. I interpreted that he avoided involving himself in work as well as in his treatment in order to avoid the anxiety that comes with it.

"What am I so terrified of?" he questioned. He then reported memories of his fouling up because of his fear of putting himself on the line, which left him feeling sad about any achievement. He felt small, thin, poor and insignificant. His parents saw the world as frightening. His family, poor in both money and spirit, conveyed the message that it was impossible for him to succeed. The father was a kind of self-centered, helpless dreamer. "Father avoided me; mother overwhelmed me. Even if I did my best, I got a negative reaction; but I never tried my hardest; I became a cautious, afraid, conventional complier."

For a long time he had wanted to write an article on a subject that interested him greatly, computers, but he had kept putting it off, procrastinating, rationalizing that he would get around to it someday. I pointed out this avoidance and said that the price he had to pay was that he never got the pleasure of having written the article. He then tried to write the article, which mobilized all his defenses against individuation. He described trying to do it, first holding back emotional commitment and then becoming overwhelmed with anxiety that he would fail and finally just dropping the effort and going on to something else.

He became aware that his work schedule was filled with obsessive detail based on fulfilling obligations rather than on what he wanted to do. He began efforts to change. He became aware for the first time of reading from curiosity and interest rather than from obligation: "Life had all been a matter of homework; education for me was a smoke screen to hide avoidance of commitment to myself. I'm excited about doing what I want to do, but another part of me won't give in; there is a break on it; I'm afraid to believe in it, afraid a disaster will occur."

He reported: "My wife has disdain for my lack of confidence in myself. She attacks me. Looking back on my life I see that my lack of confidence led me to avoid taking risks, feeling pessimistic, dissatisfied and unhappy. Is it me or is it my wife?" I suggested that the lack of confidence seen in his behavior with his wife promoted her disdainful attitude (his wife was disappointed and disillusioned by his excessive pessimism).

I pointed out to the patient that his withdrawing part-unit projections—i.e., if he individuates, it will be a disaster—seemed to exclude reality entirely; that if he asserted himself, he considered no other consequence than disaster. I pointed out that even though the treatment had been going fairly well, he still withheld full commitment. He responded: "Whatever I do will turn out badly. I limp through life, avoiding activities, not supporting myself, my own ideas. I'm constantly self-critical and allow my wife to be condescending."

He then reported that, although he seemed to be avoiding life less, he was more depressed, feeling alone and scared, attempting to comply more with his wife and wondering why. He then recalled a crucial period in his life between ages eight and ten, prior to which he felt quite fresh and alive. Between eight and ten, he got depressed, used illness to avoid school, felt disinterested in everything, had no friends, and performed poorly in school. All this occurred after he moved to a different city where he had no friends.

His depression, stimulated by the analysis of his avoidance, continued, as he became more and more aware of the difference between "what I know and my negative projections about it. I'm beginning to see how pervasive the latter are and how they override reality." The patient was beginning to integrate my confrontations about challenging the projections: "I see how I substitute one negative projection for another."

This integration triggered his withdrawing part-unit, which he projected on me: "I'm angry with you because life is not working out better, as you promised. Why don't you talk more; you're withholding from me, taking me for granted; this is all very hard work." He again reported his wife being critical, attacking him, putting him down, his becoming angry but not making any efforts to set limits. As he struggled to control the avoidance, to individuate and to deal with his compliance, the withdrawing-unit projection took specific form with: "I'm constantly afraid you will withdraw. If I open up and let you in, you'll trick me and not be there; if I do assert myself, it will be so horrendous, you'll withdraw. This feeling has the strength of a conviction."

This led him back to a memory of when, at age six, his vision of the world changed from one of bright colors to being gray. He became terrified. He recalled an incident (age five) when he was terrified by his mother's absence. He reported that his mother never lost any love over him, and she didn't like him now either; that she still couldn't recall essential facts about his life and continued to call him "Michael," although he preferred "Mike."

"Mother has a hold on me to this day. I still don't understand; I still get caught in her ideas. She was disappointed in my two divorces; she supported my wives." I suggested that mothers most often supported their own sons. "She was disappointed at my becoming a writer." These few efforts at coming to grips with a reality perception of the mother led to intense guilt in the next session, where he questioned whether or not he painted her too black. I noted the paradox—how much he wanted to avoid disappointing her, although she never stood up for him and was always tough, critical, and dogmatic.

"She treated me as a bad child. She blamed me for her miscarriage and when she had another child that died after childbirth, I moved out of the house in a panic, because I didn't want to have to handle her depression. I wanted a mother with an image of kindness and one who was interested in me, but where did it come from? She was never that way with me. I created a fictional figure" [a rewarding unit]. He reported feeling angry and cheated, that he constantly tried to get his mother's approval but never got it. He actually went to a professional school to please her, but she was most interested in grades. He constantly buried his anger to seek her approval and, unfortunately, bought mother's view of himself: "Why did I buy her view of me? She was such a powerhouse, I felt trapped by her and so scared as a kid that I played it safe. I wanted a powerful man to be a bulwark against my mother, but my father was never there." When he talked about mother or his prior wives or present wife, I pointed out that he tended to become circumstantial, lose focus and stress mostly his own negative sides. "I expected it to be my fault and be attacked for it. When I object to anything about a woman, I say to myself that it is petty and tell myself to forget it."

The patient asserted himself with his wife about her using him as an emotional target: "I'm moving towards a new alignment. I have more confidence in myself, yet I can see myself slip back into it. It is because of the doom and gloom projection." Occasionally, his individuation would shine through these negative projections: "The thought of being able to do what I want is exhilarating to me but makes me anxious. I constantly subject my own ideas to whatever objections or criticisms I raise and then give up. I'm afraid to run my own life. As I begin to change my own schedule and do more of what I want, it's much more enjoyable, but I can't seem to face the world on my own. I give up and go back to holding on. Whenever I was away from home I was happier, but I always went back. I always took the line of least resistance and let other people take over. I was always intimidated and awed by authorities. I have to start taking charge and do what I want. It's such hard work." I pointed out to him that his attitude toward work was like a prisoner on a rock pile, whereas what he actually was considering doing was exactly what he wanted. A short while later he reported: "I can now see my way clear to doing what I want—I have never been so clear about my own projections and my own avoidance. Things are falling into place mostly around my work, and I feel more in control of my life than I ever have—and I am amazed at my self-deceptions."

To recapitulate the patient's progress to this point: First the patient's avoidance mechanisms were confronted. He integrated the confrontations and began to make efforts to overcome the avoidance and individuate, but then he gave up to avoid coming to grips with the withdrawing part-unit doom and gloom projections. When this was confronted ("Why don't you challenge the projections?"), he again returned to individuation, but then he projected onto me the withdrawing object relations unit. Finally he began to examine and set limits to his projection. However, throughout this period he made at best sporadic efforts to assert himself and set limits with his wife. As his individuation efforts began to gain some continuity, the expected abandonment depression did not surface, because he had deposited it with his wife through his compliant behavior. In other words, he had still externalized it. His depression would not surface so that it could be pushed back into his head and worked through until he overcame the compliant behavior and asserted himself with his wife, thereby removing the withdrawing-unit projections.

He reported that he saw all women as arrogant, overbearing, unable to change, implacable, overwhelming, controlling; he said that he was afraid of all of them. He made sporadic efforts to set limits to their behaviors and then gave up. "Why am I so over-concerned about my mother and my wife's anger at me?" He reviewed some of the history with his mother and father. He reported rather blatant sexual acting-out of the father which was minimized and denied in the family. I brought this to his attention, which changed his perception for the first time: "I realized for the first time the extent of my denial about my parents." He then elaborated on his father's self-centeredness and his sexual acting-out, as well as his professional failure.

In the midst of "mounting excitement and pleasure at seeing that life can be better," the patient reported positive feelings about me, the therapist, as one of the few people who were interested in him and encouraged him to try things. However, it still made him afraid: "If someone withdraws, I feel attacked." I then pursued his wish to be taken care of through some homosexual fantasies and his wish for a father to take care of him. I suggested that he had been seduced by his first therapist, that he had traded treatment for approval.

He never saw women as caretakers. He never considered seeing a woman analyst and feared all relationships with women were sterile and not worth it. He reported that his father, in his will, had left money to his mother and brother but not to him, although he was just as needy as they. He rationalized the father's behavior, which I pointed out to him.

A good illustration of the patient's resistance is that he had a dream and then reported no free association and moved on. When I questioned him as to why, he took my question as a direction to associate and started in to do it intellectually, which I pointed out to him—he complied in order to avoid feeling.

In the setting of his brother getting into trouble with the law and the mother supporting the brother's denial, the patient's remaining fantasies about the family—father, mother and brother —collapsed, and he began to see that he sacrificed himself to gain their approval, that he could not face the way they were because it made him feel hopeless. "I kept thinking if I worked hard enough I would get their approval." My father was so afraid of life, he couldn't support me. He put me down. He never talked to me, he had no interest in me. He bragged about homosexual relations and affairs." Depression and disillusionment followed the analysis of his now frustrated fantasies about his parents, and he responded by stopping the thrust toward individuation: "What's the point— life is a wreck—I give up." Not only was he disillusioned about them, but he felt contaminated and tainted like a contagion.

As he worked this through he gradually improved and said: "Even though I have made progress, the hopelessness and despair persist and constantly tell me to give up. However, things are finally going well. I'm tougher than I used to be; I'm trying to support myself wherever I can. The repeated cycle of efforts at individuation, depression, despair and hopelessness, and giving-up was interpreted. This led to his reporting feelings of disgust and contempt and anger at himself for stalling. I pointed out that although he was aware that he sacrificed himself, he never analyzed this side, and I wondered why. To this he responded, "I don't know what to do about it." I said, "Why are you so helpless?" He replied, "The self sabotage is clear to me. I am destined to fail! There is a giant standing in the door saying that I can't go. If I'm not constantly on guard, avoidance takes over. As soon as I feel good, something destructive happens." I again confronted that he does not challenge the withdrawing part-unit projections, but has a tendency to give in, to give up on individuation to avoid his despair and depression. "I'm a prisoner of the voice, a robot, an automaton. I'm so cowed by those voices that I don't challenge them—the litany is so powerful." I pointed out that they were so powerful probably because they were not challenged.

He then challenged his wife, saying that their lifestyle enabled them to avoid each other and make no commitment to each other. The wife seemed to respond to this challenge. Then he had a dream: "I was dying, I was famous, people were taking my picture —I told my wife I wouldn't let myself die—I would gather my resources and get stronger." He free associated: "I had a fantasy of not letting myself die until my kids could take care of themselves. Is this dream about asserting myself or about my wife? My relationship to you means a lot to me. Maybe I don't want to get better because I'll have to give it up."

PRINCIPLES OF TREATMENT OF A PATIENT WITH A FALSE SELF

In the first case, Susan D., who as a child had to stimulate a psychotic mother to retain her attention and then had to comply with a severely critical and hostile father, harvested a rewarding object relations part-unit characterized by intellectualized unemotional responses to expectations, beneath which lay a withdrawing unit terribly critical about self-expression. In the second case, the guilt instilled in Michael E. by the mother for her inability to function fully as a woman could only be atoned for by meeting her expectations of being a success, again at the cost of individuation. Of course, there is more to this. For example, the latter patient had a narcissistic father and had such negative feelings about his father's narcissism that he couldn't tell the difference between healthy and pathologic narcissism.

These patients present a specific problem in psychotherapy, because they respond like chameleons, picking expectations almost out of the atmosphere in order to repeat their past in the transference to avoid individuation and separation anxiety. The therapist must be excruciatingly careful not to convey expectations by tone, word or deed, except that the patient express himself and try to understand himself; otherwise, the therapist is drawn into resonating with the projection. Of course, to a certain extent this will happen anyway, but it is terribly important that the therapist take special care to keep his therapeutic behavior within objective limits in order not to give the patient fodder for the projection.

The key to the work in the beginning of treatment is *affect*—to track and bring to the patient's attention the discrepancy between his behavior and his feeling state while setting limits to the rewarding unit projections. This inevitably leads to the triggering of the withdrawing unit, which must then also be confronted.

In the patient with the clinical false self, we see in the transference a repetition of the early interaction with the mother. The child incorporates, or swallows whole, so to speak, the maternal projection and develops object representations which are unmodified replicas. These unmodified replicas never get a chance to be reshaped by further growth, development and interaction with reality, as happens in normal development. They continue unaltered. These replicas of part-objects contain both the extraordinary hostility to the individuation and the active, responsive reward for developing a false self. It is as if, when the self began to emerge from the object, the anxiety and depression were so intense that the infant automatically and instantly dropped its individuative moves and imposed upon its individuation this internalized object, which then became a basis for all motivation for a defense against individuation as well as for adaptation to reality. This became incorporated later as his own self-image—a false self-image.

A specific and unique clinical management problem with a false-self patient is that, like a chameleon, he is tempted always to repeat with the therapist the same solution that worked earlier with the mother, i.e., to completely forgo or drop his own individuation and swallow whole what he can find or perceive of the therapist's perceptions as a new but equally foreign model to use for both defense and adaptation. As the false-self defense is being resolved, we see emerge the extraordinarily hostile and negative feelings of the withdrawing part-unit to individuation. Only when these are worked through can the real or true self emerge. From this perspective, the treatment is akin to the work of a diver who recovers an ancient object from the sea but cannot determine its true form and quality because the centuries of encrustation by the silt and flora and fauna of the ocean floor have completely covered over and obliterated its outline. Only after he has patiently and carefully removed these encrustations does the true form emerge.

To return to the classification of self-image disturbances, the poor self-image is the least severe of the three, as the patient is aware of and reports his poor self-image, his difficulty in articulating his wishes and feelings in reality and his difficulty with self-assertion.

SUMMARY

We can now add this additional vector to the psychopathology of the borderline patient: There is a self-image distortion and difficulty in identifying and activating individuative thoughts, wishes and feelings into reality, as well as difficulty with self-assertion. This aspect of the borderline psychopathology was implied in my use of the phrase "a failure to individuate," but its importance was overshadowed by the abandonment depression and the ego and superego fixation. To these must now be added and equally emphasized the parallel failures of self-expression.

II. The Borderline Personality Disorder

The purpose of this section is to bring the readers of my previous publications (83-88) and other readers up-to-date on the latest perspective on the borderline personality disorder in order to better contrast it with the narcissistic personality disorder.

The active process of clinical research entails constant reevaluations of earlier findings and ideas as some become reinforced and others are qualified. Chapter 7 presents in summary form revisions, additions and qualifications which have stemmed from reflection and study prompted by questions raised regarding the theory in the last eight years, as well as review of related studies published over the same period. These revisions are in the following areas:

(a) maternal libidinal unavailability and the borderline syndrome;
(b) rapprochement subphase of separation-individuation;
(c) rewarding and withdrawing part-unit pathologic ego alliances;
(d) the development of the borderline after the stage of separation-individuation;
(e) use of the therapist's technique of confrontation;
(f) cautions regarding clinical research.

Chapter 8 presents the case histories of three borderline patients, one upper-level and two lower-level, along with an analysis of their intrapsychic structure, as a prelude to Chapters 9 and 10, which describe in detail the vicissitudes of the intrapsychic structures in the treatment of these patients. Chapter 9 emphasizes the use of confrontation to establish a therapeutic alliance, while Chapter 10 focuses on the therapeutic techniques required to maintain these patients in the working-through phase of treatment. Although some of this material was taken from previously published papers, it has been extensively revised and updated; also, completely new case illustrations have been added.

Chapter 11 describes the importance to successful treatment of the patient's mastery of the talionic impulse. Chapter 12 presents problems involved in the termination of treatment.

7

A Revision and Update
of Developmental
Theory

In my initial publications between 1972 and 1976 (83-86, 88), I emphasized the nurture side of the equation, suggesting that the mother of the borderline child was borderline herself and required the child to resonate with her projections through regressive behavior to defend her against separation anxiety. She withdrew her supplies because the child was individuating and exposing her to separation anxiety. This withdrawal produced the abandonment depression and the developmental arrest in the child. This view derived from 1) the observation of many, many borderline adolescents and their mothers in analytic psychotherapy for several years; 2) family interviews with borderline parents and their adolescents; and 3) treatment of borderline mothers in my own practice. The evidence seemed at the time and still seems persuasive.

Although this view met with general acceptance, the question was raised that the concept of the borderline mother as an etiologic and psychodynamic force was too narrowly drawn. Re-study of the issue in the light of these reservations and of articles published in the last eight years has led to some additions to the original concept. The reasons I emphasized the role of the borderline mother were: First, the great majority of the mothers of the borderline adolescents we studied were indeed borderline—re-study of the original material confirmed that fact; second, this type of mother illustrated best the two-way, unique, specific and intimate tie between mother and child, wherein the mother required the child's compliance with her projections to defend against separation anxiety; third, this unique, specific interaction was the best illustration to confront the resistance, even among professionals, to recognizing the degree of the mother's pathology.

This view as originally stated remains unchanged as one of the possible etiological agents; however, it now requires the following addition: Contributions to the etiology may come from either or both sides of the mother-child equation—from both nature and nurture. Examples of the former would be minimal brain damage or developmental lags or disharmonies (115). As to the latter, we now see that the mother may have a disorder even more serious than a borderline syndrome, including psychosis. Mothers who are depressed or empty, as well as those who are ill or physically absent during this crucial period, contribute to the etiology.

The key issue is the mother's libidinal unavailability for the child's separation-individuation needs; the unavailability itself can be due to a variety of reasons. The child responds to the unavail-ability as an absence or withdrawal of a vital need and introjects it as a withdrawing maternal part-object. For example, whether the mother clings and rewards regressive behavior and withdraws from separation-individuation behavior or is neutral to regressive behavior but prematurely and inappropriately promotes in-dividuation because she cannot tolerate the child's dependence, the child will respond to both as failure to respond with com-municative matching and cueing to his/her unique separation-individuation needs and will introject a withdrawing object-relations maternal part-unit. To repeat, the key is the child's emotional experience of the withdrawal which he/she introjects as a withdrawing object relations part-unit. As a part of the intrapsychic structure, it may be reshaped and reorganized by later stages of development; nevertheless, with its affect of abandonment depression, it remains as the driving affective force of the disorder and can be identified as such in the transference acting-out. Thus arises the borderline triad: Separation-individuation leads to depression which leads to defense.

THE RAPPROCHEMENT SUBPHASE OF SEPARATION-INDIVIDUATION

My earlier publications did not adequately emphasize that the normal developmental vicissitudes of the rapprochement subphase, the surge of individuation accompanying the acquisition of locomotion and speech, as well as the increased awareness of the separateness from the mother which triggers the child's increased sensitivity and need for the mother, become unique vulnerabilities for the borderline child. His/her very surge of individuation, which brings with it a greater need for the mother's support, actually induces withdrawal of that support, i.e., the vital process in which he/she is engaged produces the withdrawal that arrests that process and results in the abandonment depression.

SPLIT OBJECT RELATIONS UNIT/PATHOLOGIC EGO ALLIANCES

The earlier publications emphasized only the therapeutic alliance of the pathologic ego with the rewarding part-unit. It must now be added that the pathological ego can form alliances alternately with the rewarding object relations part-unit or the withdrawing part-unit, the primary purpose of which is to promote the "good" feeling and to defend against the feeling of abandonment. Although both types may alternate in each patient, one tends to predominate.

In addition, I described the manifestations of those projections in treatment as transference. As is discussed in detail in Chapter 9, it is not transference but, more specifically, transference acting-out.

Rewarding Part-Unit/Pathologic Ego Alliance
(Internalized Defense)

When the withdrawing part-unit remains internalized and is experienced as abandonment depression, it is defended against by projection and acting-out (or externalization) of the rewarding object relations unit onto the environment. This is seen clinically in the transference acting-out by dramatic or subtle clinging, compliant behavior. The patient projects the part-object representation of the rewarding unit onto the therapist and/or a person in the environment, behaves in a compliant manner, and expects that person to resonate with the projection and provide approval and support. This promotes the denial of separateness and potentiates the acting-out of reunion fantasies, thus relieving the abandonment depression. He "feels good," but under the sway of the pathologic ego is usually found to be acting in a regressive, self-destructive manner. The prime example of this will be seen in the content of the psychotherapy, where the patient will be denying and avoiding any and all thoughts, feelings and life events that might interfere with this defense and precipitate depression. The patient will inevitably not be doing the necessary work of the psychotherapy, which essentially comes to a standstill. This latter fact the patient will deny.

Withdrawing Part-Unit/Pathologic Ego Alliance
(Externalized Defense)

When the withdrawing part-unit is externalized by projection and acting-out and, therefore, is not experienced as internal, this would be observed clinically as the distancing transference acting-out. The patient presents not compliant behavior but the projection of the part-object representation of the withdrawing unit, with its critical, hostile attitudes, onto the therapist and/or a person in the environment, resulting in various "distancing" behaviors to defend against the projected hostility: silence, intellectualization without affect, paranoid-like attitudes about the therapist's motivation, etc. The patient also will avoid and deny all the thoughts, feelings and life situations that interfere with this defense, and they will not arise in psychotherapy, bringing progress to a halt in a dynamic similar to the clinging defense. The rewarding unit remains internalized and is expressed through hidden fantasies.

A slightly different clinical picture occurs when the patient is projecting the part-self representation (usually of the WORU) rather than the part-object representation onto the psychotherapist. In this version of the acting-out, the patient acts out the role of the part-object representation of the WORU and treats the therapist as the part-self representation, thereby externalizing his abandonment depression with the same results as with the other types of acting-out already described.

LATER DEVELOPMENT OF THE BORDERLINE

As the borderline child emerges from the separation-individuation phase with a fixated intrapsychic structure that will persist and dominate his adaptation, he enters the phallic-oedipal phase when, all too often, a scapegoating occurs at the hands of the parents that is as distorted as the earlier scapegoating (79). This results in a condensation of pregenital and genital conflicts and a premature development of oedipal conflicts that, although an effort is made to escape, results generally in some form of sado-masochistic sexual adaptation which reflects the overriding influence of the earlier level of aggression and conflict. The earlier separation-individuation conflict has now possibly been reshaped by the efforts at resolution of the condensed oedipal conflict which overlaps it. The latency stage is characterized by failure to sublimate and learn the necessary adaptive skills, and adolescence as a developmental stage is regressively avoided or often produces a symptomatic episode through the patient's inability to free himself or herself from the infantile object.

CONFRONTATION

This therapeutic technique is so vital to the success of the treatment of the borderline and there is so much confusion regarding it that it is discussed once again below.

The poor reality perception of the borderline patient, together with the degree to which primitive pathologic defenses—splitting, avoidance, denial, acting-out, projection, clinging, projective identification—result in the further obscuring of reality, leaves the borderline patient at a great disadvantage in adapting to reality. In addition, the aim of his/her repetition compulsion is not to master conflict, as in the neurotic, but to avoid separation anxiety and abandonment depression. Consequently, he/she cannot perceive the reality unaided, and the repetitive compulsion will not impel him to bring the conflict into treatment. The therapeutic confrontations lend to the patient the therapist's reality perception and thereby help him/her to start to repair this defect through identification.

The initial objective of the therapist is to render the functioning of the split object relations unit/pathologic ego alliances ego-alien by means of confrontation, i.e., confronting the defenses of the borderline triad.

Confrontation has two meanings: to oppose or challenge and to cause to meet or bring face-to-face. The first meaning implies an aggressive opposition, for example, countries opposing each other over foreign policy. The second meaning is the one implied in the use of the word as a therapeutic technique: bringing the patient face-to-face with the denied destructive aspects of his behavior and feeling states. It must be done intuitively and emphatically and must "fit" the clinical material the patient presents. It requires that the therapist confront from a neutral, objective, emotional stance because it is clinically indicated, not out of anger or from his own personal emotional needs, i.e., to be aggressive and assertive, to direct, control or admonish the patient. When done from the latter motives, it becomes self-defeating. The confrontation, if successful, causes the patient anxiety, and to defend against it, he often projects. The therapist who is confronting out of his own needs provides fodder for the patient's projections; i.e., the therapist is doing it because he is mad, not because it is appropriate and in the patient's interest.

The content of the confrontation differs with the two types of transference. The clinging transference calls for the confrontation of the denial of destructive behavior, usually outside the interview, but often, of course, also inside, while the distancing transference calls for the confrontation of negative, hostile projections, usually on the therapist. The latter is more difficult and must be more carefully done, particularly with those patients who use the distancing transference almost exclusively.

The confrontation, when taken in and integrated by the patient, overcomes the avoidance and denial and creates a conflict where none had previously existed. The patient now perceives the destructiveness of his behavior, and although he is tempted to continue it to relieve his abandonment depression, he recognizes that he cannot do so without being harmful to himself. This interrupts the operation of the borderline triad and leads him to control the behavior, which then activates the WORU, which in turn activates again the RORU as a resistance. There results a circular process, sequentially including resistance, confrontation, working-through of the feelings of abandonment (withdrawing part-unit), further resistance (rewarding part-unit) and further confrontation, which leads in turn to further working-through. Finally, a more or less continuous activation of the WORU occurs as the focus of the therapy concentrates through fantasies, dreams, memories and painful affects (anxiety and depression) on working-through the patient's depression at separation from the mother.

CAUTIONS ABOUT CLINICAL RESEARCH

The obscurities and ambiguities of the clinical picture of the borderline and narcissistic disorders have led us to repair to theory in order to understand these conditions. Despite the fact that theory greatly helped to accomplish this task, it is important to understand some of the complex issues involved as well as the limitations of the clinical application of developmental theory.

The theory derives from two sources: child observation research and reconstruction from the analysis of borderline and narcissistic adults and adolescents. The adults are often, in addition, seen in their role as parents, which sheds more light on the parents' emotional input into these disorders.

Child Observation Research

The early mother-child interaction is both affectively extremely complex and fateful for later development. The natural observation of children by analytic observers as they grow through these early stages of development has produced dramatic breakthroughs in our knowledge of the contributions of these stages to early ego development. This, in turn, has provided the background for and made possible the elaboration of theories of how difficulties in these early stages can result in borderline and narcissistic disorders.

However, a number of cautions must be kept in mind in applying these findings: They are based on assumptions from observations of the behavior of infants in preverbal stages when they cannot tell the observer what they feel. Therefore, doubt must always remain as to the precision of these assumptions. Nevertheless, they do not violate what we know of human functioning from other sources, and they look from the outside to reflect what we know from the study of children and adolescents of older ages to be relevant to what is going on inside. Beyond that, in the infant, unlike the adult, feeling states tend to be experienced and expressed more directly and openly (95).

In addition, it is impossible to predict the future course of a given childhood constellation because of the complexity and variety of the forces that will be later involved. For example, following the principles of epigenesis, development is viewed as proceeding from shifts in the patterning of already existing structures, not just the addition of new structures, i.e., synthesis, progressive organization and reorganization and change of function whereby old behaviors acquire new functions (42). Since at a given point in time one cannot anticipate the consequences of these later developments, the eventual outcome of a given constellation has to remain in doubt.

Reconstruction in Analysis of Borderline and Narcissistic Adults and Adolescents

It is as difficult to reconstruct the past in an analysis, with all the distortions of memories and gaps, as it is to try to predict the future from a given childhood constellation.

Difficulty in the earlier phases of development affect the shape and structure of later phases, and the later phases in turn reshape and restructure the earlier. For example, rapprochement fixation of the borderline affects the shape of oedipal stage and vice versa. In addition, multiple memories of a similar kind are "telescoped" so that it becomes difficult to trace the precise time of an event's occurrence; one configuration may become condensed with another, early memories affect later ones, later affect the recall of earlier ones, and earlier memories may exert their effect on later by their form only and not their content (42). Nevertheless, what one sees and must decipher in the patient is a fantasy determined by a blending of what actually happened plus the subjective impact and intrapsychic elaboration of the experience at the time, plus the transformation these feeling states may have undergone in the course of subsequent developments.

The Clinical Picture:
The Borderline Triad

This chapter introduces two borderline cases, demonstrating how the intrapsychic structure is derived from the patient's clinical picture and how the borderline triad operates. Fred and Leslie are lower-level borderline patients. The vicissitudes of the clinical manifestations of the intrapsychic structures as they ebb and flow in treatment and are dealt with by the therapist in the testing and working-through phases will be demonstrated in Chapters 9 and 10 for these two patients, as well as for Ann B., whose history was presented in Chapter 2 (pp. 33-37).

FRED F.

Chief Complaint

"Life had no meaning for me." Fred, 20, had dropped out of college because of severe depression and a work inhibition; he couldn't study or even think. He reported, "I suddenly realized that I had no motivation to study; I began to wonder why I was at school. Was it just because I was conditioned to go? I had no goals. . . . I looked at myself even more deeply, realizing I was so sensitive that I considered everything an insult. I tended to look at things from other people's points of view rather than my own.

"Even sex was not right. I could sleep with a girl, but it had no meaning for me except the physical release. I couldn't look a girl in the eye and be open with her. I've never been able to be myself. I thought that the restrictions of the previous college had prevented me and that I could be more open, more myself at this new school, but I found out that I couldn't. I realized all of this, became terribly depressed and decided I could no longer go on."

Fred then further described the onset of his overt difficulties several years earlier, as well as (what is so common for the borderline) previous interest in psychotherapy that was frustrated by his own ambivalence or by his parents.

"The more I thought about it, the more I realized the trouble went back to my junior year in high school when I first met a girl and began to have a lot of trouble with my mother, who objected to the girl. I also disliked the discipline at the school. I lost my motivation to study and my marks went down. I knew I should leave; I became negative and angry. I began to cut classes. I had been captain of the tennis team and dropped out when I realized that I did it because I felt I owed it to everybody else and not for myself. I wanted treatment at that time, but my mother was against it. As a result, my marks were poor in my senior year, and since no good college accepted me, I had to take my last choice."

Past History

Fred gave a very sketchy past history, saying that he could not remember much before age 11. The third of three children, he recalled that the family was fragmented, mother and father never being home together, never doing anything together. He could recall no love or warmth at home. He "obeyed mother" until he was a junior in high school. He had no difficulties in grammar school or early high school, until he came into conflict with his mother when he started dating in the eleventh grade.

Family History

Mother was domineering, never wrong, never able to admit faults or accept criticism. Father was a successful businessman who worked all the time, was rarely home, was quite dependent on his own family. Although "kind," he tended to put trouble out of his mind and to avoid any conflict with the patient's mother. Fred recalled that until high school he did exactly what his mother and father wanted. If she gave him trouble about being out of the house or being with other boys or girls, he would stop seeing them.

He was close to his sister, age 28, who was also in psychotherapy for severe difficulties, having developed no career of her own and no continuous relationships with men.

The Intrapsychic Structure

Analysis of the patient's split object relations part-units revealed the following structure: a withdrawing part-unit with a part-object representation consisting of a condensed image of both the attacking mother and the withdrawing father; the predominant affect of abandonment depression; the part-self representation of a person who had caused the abandonment, who had leprosy, was no good, inadequate, "crazy" and "bad." The rewarding part-unit consisted of a part-object representation of a father who rewards passivity with the affect of feeling "good" and the part-self representation of an obedient child. This unit was allied with the pathological ego's use of avoidance, inhibition and passivity with denial of reality in pursuit of the wish for reunion.

The alliance between the rewarding unit and the pathologic ego operated as follows: If the patient gave up his self (own thoughts, feelings, motivations and assertiveness) and submitted passively, the father would love him and take care of him. Activity and aggression, especially anger, must be inhibited along with all associated activities such as learning, as they would activate the withdrawing part-unit.

LESLIE G.

History of Present Illness

Leslie, 19, was a freshman in college who had been an outstanding high school student and who had subsequently dropped out of college because of depression and "panic." The mother, on the one hand, pushed the patient for academic success, while on the other hand she infantilized her and overstimulated her with stories of her sexual difficulties with the father. The sister, age 20, a sophomore in college who was capable, outgoing, and charming, was in conflict with the patient. A brother, 16, a junior in high school, was active and assertive; he had many outside interests and was the apple of the father's eye. The patient envied his position in the family.

The patient's father had had recurrent depressions and had an explosive temper. Throughout the patient's childhood, the father had behaved as a dependent child in his relationship with the mother; he had openly attacked the patient for her "childhood inadequacies" but had envied her achievement. The major role confusion within the family found the mother playing the role of the father's mother and demanding that the patient not only submit to the father's attacks but also serve in the role of her own (the mother's) mother.

Past History

Leslie was the second of three children; early development was reported as normal until the age of three, when she had attacks of asthma that would occur frequently when she developed infections; she often had to stay home from school because of them. She went to local private schools, where she was a very good student and described herself as being "a docile kid." At age three, when the asthma began, she had temper tantrums for a year.

She managed grammar school without further difficulty from the asthma until age 11, just prior to going on her first trip to camp, when she had a severe attack and became an invalid. She missed the seventh and eighth grades because of the asthma and had to remain immobilized at home with her mother. During this period she used fantasy extensively for gratification.

She returned to school in the ninth grade, felt she had lost out socially because of the two-year absence but was able to get into some school activity such as managing the paper and being in a play, and she continued to do quite well academically. "I could push myself to achieve, but I never enjoyed it." Later in treatment her extensive sadomasochistic fantasy life at this time came out, but initially she reported very little dating and very little sexual interest or activity.

Intrapsychic Structure

The patient's withdrawing maternal part-image was that of a mother who exploited her and who was deliberately cruel and enjoyed the patient's helplessness and dependency; the associated affect included abandonment depression and the fear of engulfment; the part-self image was that of being inadequate, worthless, guilty, an insect, a bug. The patient harbored cannibalistic fantasies and fears throughout childhood; in the fantasies she was at times the victim and at other times the cannibal. The rewarding maternal part-image was that of a strong, idealized ("all-good") mother who would save her from death; the associated affect was that of feeling "good," and the part-self image was that of a helpless, clinging child.

The Borderline Triad

The pathological ego's defenses consisted of avoidance of individuation, denial of separation, acting-out through clinging and helpless behavior, the RORU/pathologic ego alliance. The poor reality perception of the pathologic ego with its pursuit of pleasure led to an extensive fantasy life which expressed the affect of both the part-units.

Chapter 9 will describe the initial resistances presented by each of the patients described here and detail the psychotherapeutic techniques used to deal with these resistances in order to establish a therapeutic alliance.

9

Therapeutic Alliance, Transference Acting-out, Transference

The therapeutic alliance can be defined as a real object relationship which is conscious and in which both patient and therapist implicitly agree and understand that they are working together to help the patient mature through insight, progressive understanding and control (32, 88, 126, 128). It is based upon the capacities of the patient and the therapist to maintain a real relationship with each other as completely separate figures—whole objects with both positive and negative attributes. As a precondition for psychoanalysis, it represents an achievement in psychotherapy with the borderline.

In contrast, the transference relationship is not conscious, and the therapist is utilized not as a real object but as a displaced object upon whom is projected unresolved infantile fantasies (83, 88, 126, 128). The transference relationship, however, also requires

146

the capacity for whole object relations—for how can the patient know he is displacing feelings onto an object unless he is able also to recognize the independent existence of that object?

In psychoanalysis the therapeutic alliance forms the framework against which the fantasies, memories and emotions evoked by the transference are measured, contrasted, interpreted and worked through. The patient's awareness of the real object relationship— the therapeutic alliance—forms the essential background against which he can evaluate his displaced unresolved infantile fantasies (108).

An important contribution to the capacity for a therapeutic alliance is made by a successful resolution of the separation-individuation phase of development, where there has been encouragement of the child's efforts toward separation-individuation (36a, 64-78, 80-82, 86, 88). A relationship of mutual trust and understanding evolves with the mother in which the inevitability of life's limitations, frustrations and disappointments is understood and accepted. This early trust in the mother forms the essential beginning of the framework for the later therapeutic alliance. There will be additional inputs into this framework at each subsequent stage of development, but this forms the core.

The capacities which emerge from the ego development that flows from this early trusting relationship are also prerequisites for a therapeutic alliance: the capacities to tolerate anxiety and frustration, to accept certain reality limitations and to use an observing ego to distinguish between fantasy and reality (122-124, 126, 127).

The separation-individuation failure and resultant developmental arrest of the borderline result in emotional capacities for both a therapeutic alliance and transference—in the strictly defined sense—which are weak and fragile at best. There is little basic trust. The borderline patient does not relate to the therapist as a real, whole object, both positive and negative, but as a part object, either positive or negative, as I shall describe in more detail later. The capacity to tolerate anxiety, depression and frustration is limited; the capacity to perceive, let alone accept, reality limitations is minimal, as is the ability to differentiate between past and present, reality and fantasy, and mature and infantile aspects of mental life. Furthermore, the observing ego routinely loses its observing distance under separation crises and temporarily ceases to function therapeutically (29, 31, 50, 83, 88, 96, 126, 128).

Therefore, at the outset of therapy there is at best a brittle and fragile therapeutic alliance, so that the first, as well as a continuing, goal of the psychotherapy is to establish, strengthen and maintain a therapeutic alliance. However, this alliance will routinely, inevitably and repetitively suffer transient breakdowns whenever the patient is exposed to sufficient separation anxiety. Nevertheless, these breakdowns, properly managed, can lead the patient to understanding and mastery of his separation-individuation problem.

Since there is no transference in the strict whole-object sense of the term, what does exist? Rather than coin a new term with all the handicaps which that implies, let us call it "transference acting-out."

Freud on Transference Acting-out and Working-through

It is first necessary to review briefly the essentials of the relationship between transference acting-out and working-through which were so clearly described by Freud (22). To adapt this brilliant discussion to the borderline patient we have only to substitute the words transference acting-out for the phrase "expressing what is forgotten in behavior," splitting for repression, and confrontation for interpretation.

Freud highlighted the following: The patient remembers nothing, but expresses it in action. He/she reproduces it not in memory but in behavior. He/she repeats it in his transference acting-out. The compulsion to repeat an action which replaces the impulse to remember is activated in treatment through the transference relationship. The repetitive compulsion to act is curbed and turned into a motive for remembering by the handling of the transference (in the borderline—confrontation of transference acting-out). The repetitive compulsion then gets full play in the transference and in the therapeutic interview via thoughts, feelings, fantasies and memories. Repetitive reactions in the transference evoke affects which, when not discharged by acting-out, lead to the awakening of memories, setting the stage for working-through.

One must allow the patient time to get to know the resistance of which he/she is ignorant, to work it through, to overcome it. Only by living the resistances through in this way will the patient be conscious of their existence and power. It is an arduous task for the patient and a trial of patience for the therapist. Theoretically, one may correlate the working-through with the "abreaction" of quantities of affect pent up by repression that has been manifested in hypnosis.

A DEVELOPMENT PERSPECTIVE

The borderline transference is not simply transference but transference acting-out, which consists of the alternate activation and projection upon the therapist of each of the split object relations part-units. During those periods in which the patient projects the withdrawing part-unit (with its part-object representation of the withdrawing mother) onto the therapist, he perceives therapy as necessarily leading to feelings of abandonment, denies the reality of therapeutic benefit, and either continues to act out the WORU or activates the rewarding part-unit as a defense. When projecting the rewarding part-unit (with its reunion fantasy) onto the therapist, the patient "feels good" but, under the sway of the pathological (pleasure) ego, is usually found to be acting in a regressive, self-destructive manner. Both, however, represent forms of transference acting-out—an instant replay—in which the therapist is treated not as a real object upon whom infantile feelings are displaced, but as if he actually were the infantile object. It differs from a transference psychosis in that the patient has the capacity to distinguish between his projection and the reality of the therapist when it is brought to his attention.

Therapeutic Alliance

The patient begins therapy feeling that the behavior motivated by the RORU and WORU alliances with the pathologic ego is ego-syntonic. It makes him feel good; he is unaware of the cost to him of his denial of the reality of his self-destructive behavior and distorted attitudes.

These distinctions between the therapeutic alliance—the real object relationship—and transference—the unconscious transfer of feelings from important persons from the past onto the therapist, recognizing all the while his independent existence—and transference acting-out—the instant replay with the therapist of feelings from important persons from the past without being aware of his independent existence—are of profound importance in treatment of the borderline, since the initial and continuing goal is to convert the latter, i.e., the transference acting-out, into the former, i.e., therapeutic alliance and transference, by confrontation.

The initial objective of the therapist is to render the functioning of this alliance ego-alien by confronting its destructiveness, either the denied, destructive behavior of the RORU alliance or the distorted attitudes of the WORU alliance. Insofar as this promotes the patient to control the behavior, the withdrawing part-unit (WORU) becomes activated or contained and experienced, which in turn reactivates the original alliance, with the appearance of further resistance. There results a circular process, sequentially including resistance, confrontation, working-through of the feelings of abandonment (WORU), further resistance (RORU) and further confrontation, which leads in turn to further working-through.

In those cases in which the circular working-through process proves successful, an alliance develops between the therapist's healthy ego and the patient's embattled reality ego; this therapeutic alliance, formed through the patient's having internalized the therapist as a positive external object, proceeds to function counter to the alliance between the patient's rewarding part-unit (RORU) and his pathological (pleasure) ego, battling with the latter for control of the patient's motivations and actions.

Since borderline transference acting-out is a projection of the already well-entrenched and active split object relations part-units, it does not require a period of regression in therapy to be activated but is active at the very beginning. In addition, the separation-individuation failure leaves the borderline patient with an idiosyncratic sensitivity to the unconscious of others, particularly their rewarding and withdrawing responses (99). Combined with poor reality perceptions, this can lead to some surprising and bizarre-seeming responses to the therapist very early in therapy.

There is a reciprocal relationship between the patient's emotional investment in the rewarding unit/pathological ego alliance for the relief of separation anxiety and abandonment depression and his investment in and use of therapy and the therapist for those purposes. At the outset he resists the latter, because it means giving up the former and bringing on the feelings of abandonment. The more he invests in the therapist as a real object, the more he turns to therapy to work through his feelings of abandonment rather than to the rewarding unit/pathologic ego alliance to relieve them. The therapist's confrontation of the destructiveness of the projections of the two part-units and his support of separation-individuation facilitates this transfer of emotional investment from the rewarding unit to the therapist.

It is necessary for the therapist to patiently, consistently confront the patient with the regressive, destructive behavior associated with the rewarding part-unit projection and the distortions of reality involved in his withdrawing part-unit projection, i.e., the patient's distorted perception that a real therapeutic alliance or involvement in therapy is equivalent to the withdrawing part-unit feeling state of being engulfed or abandoned.

At the same time, the therapist demonstrates by actual behavior with the patient the necessity, function and value of trust in the therapeutic relationship. Only when this task is accomplished will the patient be willing to forego his lifelong reliance on the rewarding part-unit/pathological ego alliance for security and instead substitute the therapeutic alliance and therapy. This momentous turning point in therapy is often symbolized by the patient's identifying the now ego-alien aspect of the old rewarding part-unit/pathologic ego alliance by a disparaging nickname, e.g., "creep," "queer," "baby," "devil."

THERAPEUTIC FRAME OR SETTING

Before illustrating how the first or testing phase of treatment is managed in order to promote a therapeutic alliance, a few words are in order about the therapeutic setting or frame—all those practical arrangements necessary to conduct the treatment, such as time and place of interview, length of interview, fee, policy for lateness, cancelled appointments, vacations, etc., as well as the accidental and incidental events that can occur during the course of treatment.

Prominent among the borderline patient's motivations for coming to treatment are the wish to receive (in fantasy) the supplies and support he was deprived of in childhood, i.e., not to take full responsibility for himself and his feeling states to avoid the depression this entails, or, if not, to be able to express all those negative feelings he had had and suppressed as a child at the frustration of this wish. His acting-out implements these goals by attempting to induce the therapist to resonate either with his RORU (and provide the fantasy supplies) or his WORU (and provide a convenient target for his rage). It is vital for the therapy, however, that the therapist maintain his therapeutic neutrality and objectivity and implicitly expect the patient to assume responsibility for himself. The therapist must avoid being drawn into resonating with either the RORU or WORU. These seemingly opposed motivations set the stage for the inevitable minor skirmishes around practical arrangements that can occur at the beginning of treatment. When not managed properly, they produce "loopholes" or "leaks" in the structure of the therapeutic setting or frame which promote usually hidden or unnoticed regressive transference acting-out. The transference acting-out becomes "institutionalized" into the regular, recurring frame of the therapy where, unacknowledged, it forms a powerful resistance that even the most skillful and dedicated therapist cannot overcome. Once the therapist has altered his stance of objectivity and neutrality by overtly behaving in a manner that resonates with a resistance, he has lost his most powerful tool, which is a precondition for being able to analyze that resistance, i.e., his therapeutic objectivity.

These patients' persistent, dedicated, artful and insidious efforts, pressed with such fervor and flavor of reality, often catch therapists in what they feel is a conflict between the need to maintain a therapeutic objectivity and their wish to offer patients humane consideration and not to be harsh or punitive. This feeling is generally not a true conflict but an expression of the fact that the therapist has already been caught up in the patient's projections onto the reality of the therapeutic setting. I shall cite a few clinical examples from therapists I have supervised before discussing in more detail the various practical issues themselves and how they should be managed.

An otherwise excellent, well-trained analytic therapist, overwhelmed by the acting-out demands of a hysterical borderline patient, reports in supervision that the patient's incessant demands, both through behavior on the couch and phone calls at night asking for advice and suggestions, were too much for her to manage. Over a number of months of supervision, the therapist gradually began to set appropriate limits to the patient's behavior, and the patient began to respond. However, after about six months of supervision once a week, while we were trying to puzzle out why progress had not continued, the therapist announced out of the blue that the patient had not paid her bill in four months; besides that, the therapist had made a special and unnecessary arrangement to see this patient at a reduced fee.

Another therapist, after he had changed the location of his practice to a quite-distant town a number of years previously, was contacted by one of his old patients for treatment. He had felt himself to be somewhat inadequate in the prior course of treatment because he was finishing his training.

After a consultation with the patient, he said that the patient required treatment twice a week, and he lived too far away for it to be practical. He therefore referred the patient to another therapist in the patient's home town. The patient called back to say that nobody would do but this therapist and that she would just have to make the long trip.

The therapist agreed and even went beyond that: Rather than see her for two individual sessions a week, he made "a special arrangement" with her for one double session a week. Further inquiry into the situation revealed that he also had unnecessarily reduced her fee. In supervision the therapist reported that he found himself constantly thinking about this patient, feeling that he was not doing enough and should be doing more for her.

A careful analysis of the patient's development revealed that the patient had, in fact, functioned as the mother of her own mother, that she was projecting this image of herself on the therapist, playing the role-image of the mother herself and demanding that the therapist take care of her as she had taken care of her mother. My confrontation of the therapist's countertransference led to a good deal of anxiety and resistance before it was finally resolved by him.

These errors in maintaining the reality of the therapeutic setting are quite common and include the following:

1) unnecessary changing of the time or the hour to suit the patient's elective convenience, e.g., the patient wants to attend some recreational event that occurs at the usual interview time;
2) adding on to the end of the hour if the patient is late;
3) not requiring the patient to take responsibility for cancelled sessions or missed sessions;
4) not adequately investigating the patient's financial condi-

tion and, consequently, setting fees which are unrealisti-
cally low;

5) spending too much time on the phone or allowing phone
   calls at inappropriate hours;

6) seeing patients who are on drugs or are intoxicated;

7) not investigating and requiring that the patient pay the
   bill on time;

8) being drawn into unnecessary conversations around the
   end of the interview;

9) not starting interviews on time and ending them on time;

10) calling adult patients by their first names.

Even the most skilled therapist's vulnerability to these provo-
cative patients will vary from day to day so that it is essential for
his/her protection, as well as the patient's, that he/she develop a
series of rituals or policies to deal with these issues to avoid being
placed in the impossible position of having to decide the merits
of each individual issue with each patient as it arises. There should
be a policy with regard to lateness; the patient should be held
responsible for the time and charge if the patient is late. On the
other hand, if he is late himself, he should subtract the cost of
the time from the bill. Fees, as much as possible, should be stand-
ardized, and the patient should be expected to pay regularly each
month and be questioned if he doesn't. Interview time should
not be changed for elective reasons such as pleasure excursions.
Cancelled appointments should be charged for. A specific policy
should be laid down with regard to vacations. Patients who are
on drugs or drinking should not be seen.

If the borderline patient knows that the therapist is available
by phone, it tends to minimize his/her anxiety and thereby reduce
the impulse to call. I have never had this option abused by a
borderline patient. In addition, in the beginning it may be necessary to take phone calls at non-office hours, but this should soon
be transferred to work in the office, even if it means, as it usually
does, that the patient is indirectly transmitting his need to be
seen more often during the week. Incidentally, it must be brought

to his attention that very little productive work can be done on the phone. As long as the phone calls are not frequent enough to be intrusive, the patient whose interview is interrupted may benefit by perceiving 1) your availability when needed; 2) the reality that you do not resonate with his fantasy of belonging exclusively to him.

A policy is also necessary about seeing friends or relatives of the patient. Since the essence of the treatment is a dyadic relationship, the patient will feel that any other person he is related to whom the therapist sees is a rival for exclusive possession of the therapist. It is unwise to go beyond seeing friends or relatives in consultation and then referring them elsewhere for treatment.

A common distortion of the reasons for these policies is that they are reflections of the therapist's rigidity and his need to arrange matters to suit his own convenience. Nothing could be further from the truth. Those who understand the dynamics of transference acting-out and the vital role it plays with borderline patients can clearly see that these policies, far from being for the convenience of the therapist, actually represent a life preserver for the patient, helping him to learn how to contain his affect so that it can be made available in the sessions where he can work it through.

The following three cases illustrate the use of confrontation to establish a therapeutic alliance.

CASE ILLUSTRATIONS

Fred F.

Fred's rewarding unit based on fantasy was projected on the father, while the withdrawing unit based on reality was projected onto the therapist. The clinical content of the withdrawing unit was the patient's righteous and indignant rage at the father's failure to fulfill his part of this emotional contract. A true therapeutic alliance could not be achieved until appropriate reality limits were placed on this withdrawing part-unit projection.

Its intensity mounted to paranoid proportions, and the patient's constant temptation to get revenge on the father for his failure by acting out against the therapist and therapy always posed a threat to the continuity of the treatment and, on occasion, required seemingly extreme measures of confrontation on my part to keep the patient in treatment. This feature, which on the one hand makes an excellent illustration of the use of confrontation in establishing a therapeutic alliance, on the other hand should not be used as a guide for all cases, since it is so extreme. The intensity of the confrontation should at all times be titrated against the strength of the therapeutic alliance and the degree of separation anxiety that the patient is experiencing at the moment.

Fred acted out the part-self representation of the rewarding part-unit by massive passivity in the interviews with the expectation that I would act out the part-object representation of that unit, i.e., I would take over for him and suggest topics, direct him, give him advice, etc.

Fred's inhibition produced great difficulty in talking, and he frequently asked me what he should talk about or what he should do. When I failed to comply with these requests but instead confronted him with his passivity, the underlying angry demand of the withdrawing unit, against which the passivity was a defense, was activated, and he would become angry and accuse me of "not helping." The anger was projected and acted out by being late for interviews, by blocking, by silence, by missing interviews, by accusing me of not being interested in him, of being rigid, of having a monotonous voice, of having no affect, of being flat and bored. The financial arrangements led to critical comments about doctors being greedy and interested only in money. If my attention were to flag at all during an interview, if I were late for an interview or accepted a phone call, this would occasion an outburst of anger.

I emphasized and reemphasized the *reality* of the arrangements required to provide a framework for therapy, i.e., hours had to be arranged at regular times, as I couldn't always be available, the hour had a certain duration for both practical and therapeutic reasons, I had to charge a fee to earn a living, my need to earn a living did not conflict with my interest in his treatment.

These efforts to set reality limits were met for the most part by stony silence. My questions as to why these matters meant so much to him and why they upset him so much were summarily ignored. Fred was intensively acting out in the transference his profound disappointment and rage at the father for failing to fulfill his side of the unconscious contract. This affect was so overwhelming that there was little room left for a therapeutic alliance.

At the same time, through the operation of the splitting defense, he continued to idealize and praise his father despite blatant and obvious events which demonstrated the father's lack of interest in him. The effects of this on my feelings—countertransference and otherwise—can well be imagined. Nothing I did was any good; the father who did nothing was all-good.

Fred showed minimal ability to distinguish between fantasy and reality or between past and present on this issue. There was no past. For example, he could quite clearly describe how he had "played his role" by not confronting the mother in order to receive the father's love and support and that the father therefore owed him that support. He deserved it and had earned it with his behavior. But he could not distinguish between his feelings from the past and his feelings with me that, since he came to me for treatment, I owed him instructions and advice.

It was too early in treatment to challenge his transference acting-out beyond holding the line against his projections of anger. I would disagree with them as vigorously as necessary, saying at times that we would just have to agree to disagree, to see the issue from different points of view.

Slowly, gradually, over the course of the first ten months of therapy three times a week, my failure either to reinforce his wishes to be taken care of or to reject him because of his projected anger and my continual quiet but firm reinforcement of the limits of reality began to establish a beachhead of a therapeutic alliance, the transference acting-out diminished, and he began to try to understand his feelings. His symptoms diminished, and he returned to school.

Ann B.

Ann was seen twice a week. In the early sessions she dramatically elaborated on her panic, her symptoms, her fear of physical expression and her inability to manage. I confronted her helplessness by saying: "Why do you feel so helpless?"

This led her immediately to describe her feelings: "I don't think I can manage it myself. My mother was my worst enemy. When I was in college and calling home, she encouraged it. I was totally taken care of, overindulged. It makes it hard for me to manage myself. I never did anything completely for myself before I moved to the city. In high school I had no responsibility. This is the first job that I have had with any responsibility. I feel that now I have to show initiative and set my own goals. My life has been so structured. I never had to do it before. I never had to spend time alone. I think other people should plan for me."

Within a few sessions, confrontations caused the acute symptomatology to subside. The patient became depressed and began to talk about the difficulties between herself and her mother in a rather intellectual fashion. For example: "I dislike the idea of being responsible and taking care of myself. I don't think I can; it seems that I'll break down. I can't take the pressure. I'm an empty personality. I'd rather be an extension of someone else. I've always structured my life for someone else to do it for me."

At the time, she had a boyfriend to whom she clung and whom she used for relief of anxiety and for support. "I've never been rewarded for being an individual. I am also afraid of being depressed and alone. I never developed anything in myself on my own. I did well in college and had lots of interests, but they were all for everybody's approval."

The next level of confrontation referred to the lack of continuity between the sessions, that "the patient avoided thinking about them because they made her feel bad." She reported after one session feeling, "bad, empty, like I'm losing something, like I have to be on my own and independent, and then I get anxious and—forget about it."

Her appeals to the mother for reassurance were confronted, which encouraged her to stop calling her mother and to manage the feelings herself. Throughout these first three or four months of treatment, there was much content and symptomatology but very little genuine affect. Ann would become overwhelmed with guilt, depression and anger when she spoke about her parents with affect and would block out her thoughts in order to deal with the guilt. When the blocking was confronted, she articulated the borderline dilemma by saying: "I don't want to admit I'm competent or in control. I have to pretend I'm helpless. If I'm competent, I will be cutting mother off, or she will cut me off. I wouldn't need her anymore. She'd have no duty to perform."

As the patient continued to delve deeper into the conflict with her mother, it was necessary to confront her denial of affect in general, as well as her denial of anger and guilt at the mother. At one point, when she turned down the mother's request to spend some time with her, she said: "Mother uses me as a tool for herself. She put in my head the one thing I can't do is separate and that I would be punished for it. She was the original power. I was empty."

Following this expression, she had a nightmare that she was losing her mind, would not be able to speak, her feet would not move, that she would go crazy. Throughout this time she was clinging to the boyfriend, and it became necessary to challenge and confront her clinging, questioning why she needed him to provide her internal security, pointing out some of the destructive aspects of this behavior to their relationship. Throughout the first year of treatment, she attempted to deal with interviews by intellectualization, denial, avoidance of individuation, blocking and suppressing of affect, acting-out in the transference and through clinging with the boyfriend. The confrontation of all these defenses gradually brought about a therapeutic alliance, and she entered the working-through phase.

Leslie G.

Leslie had an extremely difficult time in therapy, beginning with the initial interview, for which she was more than half an hour late because she took the subway in the wrong direction, which indicated her ambivalence and resistance to treatment. This was expressed in the early sessions by being late for interviews regularly, by being silent in interviews, saying how much she did not want to talk. However, when she did talk, she dwelt on fantasies and dreams of being engulfed. For example, she recalled as a child being afraid of goblins under the bed, of the story of Hansel and Gretel, of Pinocchio and of Dracula. They symbolized her feeling that if she failed to comply, she would be eaten up. She talked of the fantasy of a woman fattening up a favorite doll in order to eat it, of the cyclops monster in Ulysses who roasted men over a pit.

This alternated with reports of overwhelming feelings of anger which she was unable to express, of depression and thoughts about suicide, of feelings that if she left her mother she would die, of being afraid to talk in sessions and not wanting to come to sessions. For example, she reported a dream: "I was playing with my sister. I agreed to let her kill me, then changed my mind, but my sister objected." Another dream: "I fell down. No one noticed. I had a rash. I felt very neglected and wanted to die. I felt calm and wasn't the least bit upset or confused in the dream."

During the first seven months of treatment, four times a week, she was living at home with her parents and, amidst the emotional turmoil, was trying to make up her mind whether to remain there or to move out. She was afraid of the mother's reactions if she left, as well as her own ability to cope.

The initial confrontations were directed at her being late for interviews, the paucity of affect in interviews, her silence, which was a conscious withholding, as well as her preoccupation with fantasy to avoid reality. These confrontations helped to mobilize her, and she decided after seven months to leave home and get a part-time job and live in an apartment of her own. At this point, after her first date with a boy, she had a severe panic: "I feel everyone is angry at me; I'm about to be attacked. Everyone's angry at me because I didn't want to be like my mother. I'm an insect and a bug. I'm frightened; I can no longer get along with my mother. The role I played filled her needs; it also gave me insecurity. On the other hand, I want my mother; I want to be taken care of; I can't get along without her; I can't even breathe without her. I don't have a separate existence; I feel guilty for even trying. I can't stop wanting my mother like a baby. I can't seem to make a life of my own. I don't want to talk to you, because it means growing up and being on my own. I'd rather see you as a replica of my mother and do with you what I did with her."

After a visit home, she went into a profound regression, with extreme rage and suicidal wishes. "I saw mother as the embodiment of all good things—calm, good, warm, etc., a powerful person who could take care of me. As long as I was quiet and did what she wanted, I was special. I was frightened that if she wasn't there, I would die."

As the patient further confronted the conflict with the mother in sessions and her silence disappeared, the next resistance that had to be confronted was her intellectualization with detachment of affect in order to hold on to the fantasy of reunion with the mother. This led to the patient's following fantasy: "Mother knew that I belonged to her, that I couldn't resist her; she'd have me to use and to touch." This was followed by dreams of being bitten by big spiders. She reported this conscious association: "I was afraid someone would take me over and swallow me up."

When this fear of engulfment was dealt with in the session, the patient would feel much better, her self would emerge and immediately be accompanied by a depression with longings for reunion with mother and homicidal rage. The flavor of this early period in treatment can be illustrated by the fact that after about nine months, she reported in a period of calm: "Today I felt quite normal. I wasn't even thinking about myself, taking myself for granted. I felt I could be independent. It lasted all morning, but then at lunchtime the old feelings came back. I wanted my mother. I felt depressed, angry, questioned how I could think such a thing about myself." Then she lapsed into resistance and an angry silence which again had to be confronted. When I confronted her again with her silence, she responded that she could use the talking in sessions either to try to provoke me to treat her like a child, like her mother had, or for the work of sessions, to help her grow up. After approximately a year, slowly memories began to emerge, as the psychotherapeutic alliance solidified and she entered an abandonment depression.

DISCUSSION

It is important to note that in the beginning of treatment the confrontations of the transference acting-out are limited to challenging and questioning the patient's distortions in order to set reality limits and to promote a therapeutic alliance. In many patients in confrontive therapy, these activities will constitute the bulk of the therapist's interventions. In intensive psychoanalytic psychotherapy, however, as illustrated in Chapter 10, in all these cases it becomes possible later in therapy to interpret the defensive function and the origin of the patient's transference acting-out. These interpretations must be handled with great care because, when timing and content are appropriate, they produce profound changes in the patient's intrapsychic state.

Successful therapy with the borderline patient requires both the initiation, strengthening and maturation of the therapeutic alliance and the working-through of the separation-individuation problem from the past. The demands of the former suggest that the real personality of the therapist has more effect and therefore is more crucial with the borderline than with neurotic patients. An example is the need for support of the patient's moves towards separation-individuation, which I have only barely touched on in this chapter. Ideally, the therapist should have a well developed capacity for whole object relations or, if not, he should have full awareness of his own clinging and/or distancing defenses. The requirements of this arduous but rewarding work that the therapist have both personal maturity and professional skill may help to explain many of the difficulties in learning psychotherapy of the borderline, as well as the many treatment failures. It is not so much that the patient is unable to do the work (19, 124), but that we therapists have so much difficulty providing the environment necessary to enable the patient to do the work. Our understanding of the former will always be limited until we have mastered the latter.

This chapter has illustrated the use of confrontation to establish a therapeutic alliance in three cases. Chapter 10 will illustrate the therapeutic techniques necessary to maintain these same three patients in the working-through phase of treatment.

10

Transference Acting-out and Working-through

In the initial stage of treatment as described in Chapter 9, a therapeutic alliance is gradually established by confronting the destructive aspects of the patient's transference acting-out—either the distorted perceptions involved in the projection of the withdrawing unit on the therapist or the regressive, destructive behavior associated with the rewarding unit projection.

Again, it is important to remember that the term confrontation is not used in the sense of the therapist's taking his aggression out on the patient or challenging him, but, rather, in the sense of bringing to the attention of the patient's observing ego the denied, realistically destructive aspects of his defense mechanisms, i.e., splitting, projection, projective identification, clinging, avoidance, denial and acting-out. This stage can be stormy as the tenuous and fragile alliance is repeatedly shattered each time the WORU unit is activated.

Once the patient has developed an internalized object representation of the therapist, the therapeutic alliance becomes fully activated and functions counter to the alliance between the patient's RORU and his pathological ego, battling with the latter for control of the patient's motivations and actions. As the therapeutic alliance gains the upper hand, the patient turns from his lifelong reliance on the RORU/pathologic ego alliance for relief of his separation anxiety and abandonment depression to working-through in the transference.

Entrance into the working-through phase is signaled clinically by: fewer and fewer interruptions in the continuity of the therapeutic alliance as it takes over control of behavior from the RORU/pathological ego alliance; a shift in the patient's perspective on the latter from being ego-syntonic to being ego-alien, symbolized by his assigning it a disparaging nickname, such as "creep," "baby," "monster," "devil," etc.; more realistically constructive coping behavior so that daily life crises fade from the center of the therapeutic scene and the abandonment depression deepens and is linked to the emergence of early memories. Acting-out now becomes more localized in the transference, where it must be again confronted, which again leads to more working-through. A circular process results in transference acting-out, confrontation, working-through, transference acting-out, confrontation, working-through with the debut of each new interaction in therapy. The resolution of one level of interaction through confrontation and working-through leads inevitably to more depression and then more defense—i.e., transference acting-out. The therapist must remain alert and not be lulled into a false sense of security by the transformation of one episode of transference acting-out into working-through, for as soon as that level of depression is worked through the next will again present itself as transference acting-out.

As the patient moves further into the working-through phase, the therapeutic alliance strengthens, as do the observing ego and reality perception. There is a corresponding deepening of awareness of the extraordinary ramifications of the WORU and it becomes possible to deal with transference acting-out directly by interpretation. Before shifting to interpretation, the therapist must review each episode to be sure that the transference acting-out has not overwhelmed the patient's observing ego and reality perception.

PROBLEMS IN MANAGEMENT OF TRANSFERENCE ACTING-OUT

In consultations I have done to evaluate the lack of progress of patients in psychoanalytic psychotherapy with other therapists, the single most important difficulty has been the therapist's failure to understand the psychodynamic relationship between acting-out and working-through.

For example, a 17-year-old boy had been in treatment for two and a half years, twice a week, for complaints of depression, outbursts of rage and severe compulsions that had caused him to drop out of school. Although he got along well with his therapist and his outbursts of rage had decreased in frequency, he remained depressed and compulsive and was still not back in school. Two interviews, which involved my confronting his efforts to manipulate me to ask questions, rather than to tell his own story, triggered a rage outburst that then led to his awareness that he had similarly manipulated his therapist into directing the interviews with questions, thereby reinforcing the transference acting-out of his dependency needs.

A young man, 21, with severe depression, passivity and inhibitions since the age of 15 that had led to much drug ingestion, managed to drag himself through college with psychotherapy ranging from one to three times a week. He then collapsed after graduation. He draped himself over the chair like a wet dishrag, remained silent and waited. My bringing this behavior to his attention triggered a response similar to the previous patient. He insisted that I bore the entire responsibility for the interview.

A young woman, 18, with a four-year history of anorexia nervosa, had had one year of psychotherapy, three times a week on the couch. Her analyst said little, and what little affect she had dried up. After a year of a compliant pretense at therapy, she discontinued.

A woman therapist in her mid-thirties, after 13 years of analytic psychotherapy four times a week, had a brief psychotic episode precipitated by a separation experience. This frightened her and caused her to question the strength of her character structure, as well as the effectiveness of her long course of treatment.

Two other women therapists, also in their thirties, had been in analytic psychotherapy for five years, four times a week, and felt they were "stuck" in the working-through phase, which indeed they were.

These examples illustrate how crucial it is for the therapist to understand the psychodynamic relationship between transference acting-out and working-through in the conduct of his task.

The Therapeutic Task

The need or wish to be taken care of is articulated in a fantasy which, however, remains concealed or hidden. Nonetheless, it motivates or drives the behavior of the RORU/pathologic ego alliance and can be described by various synonyms: From an instinctual point of view, it is an oral, dependent craving; from an object relations point of view, gratification of the wish for reunion expressed by clinging to the object; from a descriptive point of view, the wish to receive unconditional love or to be taken care of.

The transference acting-out of all three patients presented in the following pages consisted of efforts to manipulate me into actions which would resonate with and ostensibly gratify this fantasy and enable them to feel good, loved or special, or, barring that, have me serve as a target upon which they could externalize and ventilate their lifelong rage at the frustrations of these wishes. From the psychopathological point of view, it was seemingly a foolproof method. They couldn't lose—i.e., it enabled them to either feel loved and special or to relieve their tensions at the frustration of these wishes on the spot without having to face and accept their existence in their psyche. However, from the therapeutic point of view, they couldn't win. The therapeutic task was to set reality limits to both these projections to enable the patients to become aware of their intrapsychic function and thereby to lead the patients back to experiencing and working-through their abandonment depression.

CASE ILLUSTRATIONS

Fred F.

After a year of treatment, when Fred regressed and again began transference acting-out, I questioned the meaning of these feelings and more importantly why they had come to the fore at this moment. Fred became more argumentative and threatened to see another therapist. I held my ground and said he was entitled to see another therapist if he wished, but that if he changed therapists, he would still have to work through with the next therapist the same feelings he was going through with me. I now followed the confrontation through for the first time with an interpretation. I said that I thought these feelings actually had nothing to do with me but were related to the fact that now that he was making progress in treatment, he was feeling what he had felt at home when he attempted to express himself with his father, i.e., that the father had rejected him. He was seeing me as an exact replica of his father. I pointed out that this was not true. He was trying to replay his relationship with his father with me to avoid the pain of facing the feelings he had about his father. This interpretation was effective and led Fred to begin working through, elaborating on his lifelong search for a father, which had prevented him from "getting involved in doing his own thing."

He began to link for the first time his need for his father to his need to express himself: "I want to be myself, but I don't want to be hurt. My self wants to come out, but my need for a father overrides it." This awareness led to resistance to facing his feelings of hopelessness about his father. The resistance again was expressed in transference acting-out. "It's not my fault they threw all that crap at me. I don't ask for it. I shouldn't be suffering. If I look for reinforcement, maybe my self will come out. When I try to remember, I block out."

I reinterpreted that as he was now beginning to do better, as his self began to emerge, he turned to me as he had done with his father for reinforcement; feeling that he didn't get it, and feeling angry, he expressed the anger by blocking out and not remembering. Fred ignored the interpretation: "I'm doing everything you say. Why aren't I better?" I pointed out that he was again acting out with me this fantasy of reunion with his father, as a defense against facing his feelings of hopelessness about ever getting his father's love and support. This interpretation again relieved the transference acting-out and sent him back to working-through, with vivid memories of the father's neglect and the mother's attacks.

Ten months later, as Fred moved into the twentieth month of treatment, he was attending college fulltime and living in an apartment by himself. This progress again triggered his feelings of hopelessness and he again began to act out in the transference, as revealed by the following dream: "You displaced me with another patient, told me to control myself that I was making too much noise. I thought you had screwed me. I woke up feeling lost. You betrayed my trust. I didn't like it. My intuition was right. It makes my case hopeless." At the same time Fred reported a return of the inhibition in learning and verbalized, "I want a father, I don't want to do it myself. I want to get what I was deprived of in childhood."

I now interpreted that the purpose of the fantasy he was acting out with me was to fulfill the wish for the father that he felt he had never had and to avoid the feelings of hopelessness regarding his relationship with his real father. I noted that it arose every time he made progress and put a brake on this progress. I underlined the conflict between the defensive wish and his own growth and suggested that he would have to give up the wish and face the underlying feelings of hopelessness. Fred responded: "I felt a responsibility to my father not to get angry, not to cause a commotion." I asked what happened to the anger? Patient: "I put it on myself. Otherwise it's like hitting my father in the face." I interpreted that he was destroying himself to deal with his anger at his father.

Deciding that the time had come to deal with the splitting and projection defenses head on, I pointed out that he never had a bad word to say about his father, nor a good word to say about me —but obviously neither could be true. His father had in fact neglected him, but he had created a fantasy of a loving father on the basis of his father's verbalizations, meanwhile expressing his rage at his father's neglect by inhibition, passivity and submission, as well as projecting the rage on me and on other people, feeling they did not like him. The problem was neither other people nor me; it was his feelings about his father. I told him it was necessary to give up the fantasy of reunion and face and work out the feelings of rage at his father in therapy or else he would continue to be self-destructive. This led to further working-through of the feelings of hopelessness about the father and the mother which in turn led to further progress.

As his self emerged and became consolidated through the working-through of his abandonment depression, Fred moved into a condensed phallic-oedipal conflict manifested clinically by sadistic sexual acting-out with women. He became a "womanizer" and used women for sexual purposes and then discarded them. In the middle of working through this conflict, Fred graduated from college with honors and left to attend graduate school in another city, where he planned to continue treatment.

Ann B.

Ann began to have dreams such as the following: "A space man had two choices. He was trapped in a house, and he could either go into outer space and die or stay in the house and let people come and get him and then die." She then projected and became angry at the therapist for "making her feel these feelings. . . . I have angry feelings and then I get frightened and shake and get dizzy. I'm afraid the emotion of anger will take over. If I express it, something bad will happen to me."

Confrontation of these defenses over a period of a year led to greater individuation, which brought her face to face with her anger, which she defended against with an attack of panic and the shakes. The patient reported: "I didn't believe in my protections anymore. I started to shake and block out. I felt a craving, like heroin. I can't make it without it. I've made myself believe that if mother or you isn't there, I'm helpless. I need that like alcohol or a drug. I want to roll up in a rug on the floor like a baby. That's why I shake. I have to control that feeling. I'm afraid I'll act like a baby—either go home and drink to block it out or lie down on the floor and cry. At the same time, I am so angry at my parents."

The patient then dealt with this panic at the progress in treatment, as she had dealt with her panics as a child with her mother. In other words, she became frightened and helpless, angry and demanded that I "take care of her." The form it took was an emergency telephone call that she had taken to her bed, and she couldn't come to the interview, and I would have to come to see her because she was so upset. I asked her if she were physically ill and, when she said no, I said that I thought she should come to the sessions. She then emphasized that I didn't understand, that she couldn't move, that she was afraid her legs wouldn't walk. I recalled for her her previous similar feelings and suggested that we could not do any work unless she came. Finally she hung up on me in anger, refusing to come to the session.

At the next session two days later she reported that the panic attacks and the staying at home came from trying to suppress her anger, that she was furious at me for not taking care of her.

"But when I realized it, I calmed down, but I can't get over the feeling that if I keep stamping my foot someone will come. I feel angry, sad and hurt, but I project it on my mother. I realize she's as helpless as I feel. I feel awful when I see the anger. I get pains in my stomach and the shakes, and I can't go to work. I am dramatizing and putting on a protest, so I won't have to face the feeling of anger. I'd rather lie there and die than give her up."

At this point in treatment, the patient's symptoms dramatically subsided, much of her denial and blocking disappeared, she began to have early memories; however, she moved, not as the usual borderline patient into a working-through of the abandonment depression with the mother, but into the narcissistic identification with the father, as a defense against the borderline conflict.

"Mother never loved me for myself but only for being a child. I wanted her to love me as I am. I no longer feel I'm losing part of myself in losing mother's love. I wanted to be loved for what I am." She then recalled that, when she was eight or nine, the mother left the father and her for several weeks, and when she returned, she spent the next two years in bed.

"I felt used by mother. The only way I could be independent was to get revenge. Father was stronger, and he looked down and ignored mother and was interested in me. I decided to be like him and to do the same to mother out of anger. I wanted to madden her and make her feel left out. I do the same with you here in treatment. If you don't help me, I'll make you feel a failure as a therapist."

Working through these aspects of her borderline conflict with the mother took another year, with intimations of the narcissistic defense. Then, gradually, the narcissistic defense took over. She left her perfect boyfriend and started an affair with a self-centered, narcissistic, married man. In sessions, her behavior changed dramatically from being needy and clinging to being detached, intellectual, arrogant, devaluing of me and the treatment.

She vigorously resisted my confrontation of the part-object relation nature of the affair with all its potential risks for her. Finally, when the historical material against which the affair was an acting-out defense was broken through, her oedipal relationship with the father, she revealed that the father actually seduced her into this relationship to get revenge on the mother, that she had the same motivation but that she also was sexually aroused by the father, although there were no overt sexual activities. It made her feel extremely guilty, that she had to punish herself because she did not deserve a real relationship with a man.

In the affair with the married man, her fantasies were more concerned with getting back at the woman than with her relationship with the man. She felt compelled to do it but ashamed of herself for "being such a bad person, being so angry and so vengeful." She would have dreams occasionally of women she had previously snubbed punishing her by chopping off her breasts.

Working-through of the vengeful and oedipal aspects of the narcissistic defense resulted in her ending the affair and beginning to have relationships with a number of men who, though not married, were obviously not candidates for an appropriate, realistic relationship. Meanwhile, in sessions the theme returned to the relationship with the mother, but this time the theme changed to penis envy and feelings of women being inferior, which she had defended against through the "father-self" part of her self-image.

She developed severe tension headaches: "I don't want to give up the fantasy that father and I are allied and have a special relationship, a special attachment on which my self-image is based. Everything that makes me interesting or feel good is like father. I copied him. I built it all up. I was superior, not guilty, inferior and wrong. I'm losing a part of myself that was fun or at least felt like fun and entertaining. I have headaches and am very angry. I feel I am losing my sense of self, my sense of father-self."

This led to her anger and depression at facing the father's coldness and self-centeredness, i.e., his narcissism.

Her oedipal conflict could be condensed as follows: Mother was angry at father for his affairs outside the home and his interest in the patient. Mother set the patient up. "She used me to punish father: 'If you want her, take her.' Then mother dropped me; then I carried it out with a vengeance. If you're angry at me for taking father away, I'll really do it; I'll really show you and caricature your design. But it cost me the chance to be a real woman, carrying out this relationship with father because of how guilty it made me feel."

She felt unconsciously that she was "father's whore" and had to be punished for it. As the oedipal conflict with its guilt and shame and punishment became resolved, she finally went on to establish a relationship with a stable, solid male who was a realistic possibility and then returned in this setting to the original borderline conflict with the mother, free of the narcissistic defense, to work through her intense hostile feelings against herself, that she was worthless, despicable, etc., not lovable and not deserving of a loving relationship.

The patient's course in therapy can be tracked by observing her acting-out defenses with men, the first being the clinging relationship with the idealized male to defend against the depression with mother in the regressed state. When this was worked through, she then moved into the narcissistic defense with the father against the borderline conflict, acted out by an affair with a married man. When she worked this through, to express her disappointment in her narcissistic father's response to her, she went through the disappointment and loss and returned as her self emerged again, to work through her feelings of penis envy and then, finally, the borderline conflict with the mother, during which time she had a relationship with an appropriate man.

Leslie G.

Leslie began to recall a long period of asthma from age three to 11: "I wanted my mother; at the same time, I wanted to kill her. I hated everyone. The asthmatic attacks didn't help; I had to hold everything. I was there to take care of Mommy who had to take care of Daddy. I want to be sick all my life and never grow up. I would rather die. I wouldn't have to take care of myself or anyone else. I'm so angry I could die."

Turning to me she said: "I wish you were dead too. On the one hand, I want to be alone; on the other I want you to be my mother. I know my mother can't stand my being independent. I have to give her up and give you up. I'm furious at you. Are you helping me? Or demanding that I grow up? I hate you; I wish I were dead."

I pointed out that she seemed to see growing up only in terms of loss, and I wondered why. She responded: "Mother shared every thing. I was never alone; it was like a whole part of me would get cut off, as if mother were dead. I have always been afraid that she would leave me and die, but I get so angry, and my anger gets caught in my throat and my chest, and I want to cut them out."

A sequence evolved of the patient's presenting resistance, silence and detachment of affect which, when confronted, led to expressions of fear of engulfment, homicidal rage and suicidal depression, which in turn led, after the interview, to further emergence of the self with a greater feeling of self-confidence; this would then lead to more anxiety and more regression—for example, dreams of the family dying—and then further resistance which would then be confronted. After each confrontation, anxiety, depression and anger would resume and stimulate different historical aspects of the separation-individuation problem, from fear of engulfment by the mother to fear of abandonment by the mother, followed by fears of being humiliated and attacked by the father, introduced by the fact that, between the ages of five and 11, the father would verbally attack her.

After a little over a year, the patient was able to function in her job, was living in her apartment and described her life (or adaptation) as "going well"; "I feel good about myself. I'm not so self-conscious. I'm going to get birth-control pills and start going out with boys." She then fell silent and said that she didn't want to talk anymore and that maybe she should stop treatment. "I have a sense of self. I don't want to be a child anymore. I still feel angry and I don't want to come here."

I suggested that she seemed to be saying that if she did not require the therapy in order to just live, then she didn't require it all. I raised the possibility that she was fleeing into health in order to escape from other conflictual feelings. She replied: "I always wanted mother to share things with me, but she never did anything with me that was mine. I feel like I'm ashamed and humiliated by the fact that I still feel like an angry child and want to comply with you. I'd like to shut you out, as I did with mother in order not to feel this."

Her transference acting-out was confronted to help her face and work through this aspect of the conflict with the mother. A few months later the condensed phallic-oedipal conflict made its appearance as follows: "Now that mother is out of my head, I find my thoughts turning to father calling me a bad girl; there was a void in this relationship. Instead of wishing that I were dead, as I did before, I now feel that I hate myself."

As her interest turned toward her body-image, she recalled the many ways the mother disparaged her femininity, which led to her conflicts over how to dress and how to look and her feelings of inadequacy about being a woman: "There are two people in me: One wants to shout, fight, scream, won't work, won't cooperate; the other longs to become a woman but feels it is hopeless. Now I start to feel myself and feel bad; instead of seeing mother either taking me over or leaving me, I now see you as my father, putting me down. I feel like being nasty, willful, disagreeable, unfriendly and putting you down." As she attempted to assume her feminine-gender identity, clothing, makeup, etc., she reported the following: "I kept getting into rages at myself; I screamed at myself to stop torturing myself. The rage began because I was thinking about sex; I felt like murdering someone. It's associated with the feeling that I look awful. I realized that it was only me that despised myself, calmed down and was able to have a nice time with a girl-friend and then I had a nice sexual fantasy. Today I felt, if I could feel attractive, that would be perfect.

"In high school I felt mother didn't look at me to help me to fix myself up, because I looked so awful. I felt always like a little girl who was dressing up. Now I feel guilty, because I'm doing what mother was afraid to do—thinking of myself as feminine, attractive and letting myself be happy."

Then she acted out by picking up a man, trying sexual intercourse, found herself unable to have an orgasm and responded with feelings of weakness and rage: "I kept thinking: 'Mother wouldn't do these things. I felt so ugly today. Father always thought that I was bad and ugly.' "

The fantasies at the earlier level of being eaten were now replaced by masochistic sexual fantasies. She then proceeded at the same time into intense transference acting-out against the image of the father, which she projected; "I'm furious at you; I don't want to talk to you, to see you as my father who let me go on and did nothing to help me with my femininity."

This led to her condensed phallic/oedipal conflict, which was articulated around the fantasy: "This ugly girl falls in love with her master with no hope of his returning it, but nevertheless something identifiable is between them—something shameful and sexual. Mother didn't like the idea of my being close to father. She was the go-between; I never talked to him; I used to stay up nights hating him. I guess I do have a love for him, but I can't feel it. I wanted to be loved and be held by my father, but it was like wanting to be loved by a stranger—a terrible desire to be intimate with him. It was so painful to realize that it would never be that I shut off all feeling about him. I made a fantasy of a father who loved me. If I wanted to please him, I had to be dead. I kept wishing he loved me. The pain is very real, but I can't share it. It's my own fault for caring. Underneath, I feel angry and hopeless and despairing. I wanted to die; they didn't want me."

She elaborated further: "In adolescence I lived out this fantasy. I got so much pleasure from the fantasy that the love was returned; however, in reality my father was weak, pathetic, vulnerable, more of a little boy. He didn't exist for me."

This then led to intense affective experiences in which she had the impulse to act out the wish for her father's love in the therapy. She felt the need to sit further away, to put physical distance between us to protect herself and to look away. "I wanted a father I never had. I wanted to hold you and be close to you. I don't think my mother wanted me to have a father either. It's so frustrating; he was always there, and I couldn't get away from him, but I couldn't have him either—better off with no father at all," she said, sobbing and crying.

The complexities of this oedipal conflict, as revealed by her feelings and as acted out in the transference, are indicated in the following: "I hate you for not being my father, and I want to kill myself; I don't want to go on. I'd like to be kissed and touched and loved, and yet I feel dirty and disgusting and feel you must be angry at me because I fantasize about you. The urge is so strong, I feel raw, it hurts so much. I have fantasies of committing suicide by taking pills. All of comfort, relief and sweetness was in my father's arms, and I couldn't have any of it. I want to be hurt and whipped, have you stick nails in my sores."

As the patient works through her intense oedipal conflicts, the temptation to substitute transference acting-out for working-through is indicated by the following: "I don't want to give up the fantasy of you as my father. Talking about my sexual feelings about my father turns me on to you, and it seems uncontrollable. Then I saw you as real, which makes me want to hold on to the fantasy even more. Talking face to face ruins the fantasy and makes me angry. I feel better when I'm silent here, because I am fantasying about you as father; but on the other hand, I recognize that it is bad for me. When I come out of the fantasy, I get as mad at you for not being my father as I did at my own father, and I'd like to provoke you to fight with me so I could scream and withdraw."

This concludes the presentation of Leslie's working-through phase, although it continued on for a number of years. The conclusion is reported in Chapter 12.

DISCUSSION

These three cases illustrate that the transference acting-out (the RORU/pathologic ego alliance) is a defense against the underlying WORU part-unit with its abandonment depression and that confrontation of the former activates the latter. If the therapist confronts the transference acting-out of the RORU/pathologic ego alliance (the resistance), that which it was a defense against—the abandonment depression—will emerge and the WORU will be projected on the therapist. As this is confronted, the patient will begin to work through the depression in the interviews and the experience will be assimilated by the observing ego. The results of the separation-individuation failure will be markedly attenuated or overcome as the patient's ego, freed of the need to defend against the abandonment depression, resumes its developmental path to autonomy.

Patient and therapist alike must learn to identify, endure, cope with and eventually resolve an apparent paradox: If the therapist does his job (confrontation) and the patient begins to respond (separate and individuate), the patient feels worse, not better, i.e., more anger and depression. However, over time, as the resistances are resolved, these painful affects attenuate and give way to the patient's individuation process.

The onset of the working-through phase rekindles the patient's separation-individuation process and the therapist must be prepared in some instances for the emergence of acute symptoms such as psychotic or suicidal episodes, feelings of depersonalization or unreality, or severe paranoid projections. These events are usually transient and respond to a fuller engagement of the transference and are not by themselves contraindications to maintaining the therapeutic momentum. The temporary use of drugs and/or various environmental arrangements to safeguard the patient are warranted at these times.

The clinical examples illustrated the management of transference acting-out characterized by both clinging and distancing. In the former, the therapist must set limits to the patient's destructive actions. In the latter, the therapist must set limits not so much to the patient's actions as to the patient's projections of feelings derived from the WORU onto the therapist.

It should always be kept in mind that all patients cannot work through and therefore a thorough evaluation should be undertaken of each patient's potential for working-through.

Are the memories that are worked through memories of real events or fantasies based on feelings and distorted perceptions? In all probability they are both real events and patient's distorted elaborations of those events. It's important to keep in mind that the borderline patient is not dealing with a single memory or a traumatic event, but, rather, with an enduring pattern of interaction that not only has persisted throughout his entire lifetime but has also been internalized and become part of his psyche.

In my experience, the most therapeutic benefit is achieved if the patient can get to the bottom of what I call the tie that binds—the recognition that much of what underlies his or her pathologic behavior is the feeling that if he/she separates and individuates he/she and the mother will die. Parallel with this is the recognition of the hopelessness of the wish for unconditional love. This recognition is conveyed by a specific context of memories—which, however, focus on the meaning of events not so much in themselves but as seen within the matrix of the interaction. When these are faced in working-through, the obstructions to the individuation process are lifted sufficiently for the patient's individuation to flower. Treatment is far from finished but the psychic balance has shifted sufficiently, from the old emphasis on sacrificing adaptation to defense, to a new emphasis on adaptation and coping with reality, coupled with the use of therapy to resolve the painful feeling states that result.

11

The Role of Mastery
of the Talionic Impulse

A most important task of the working-through phase is the mastery of the talionic impulse—that deepest and most ancient of human impulses to exact revenge by taking pleasure in inflicting on others the hurt one has experienced; or as the *Bible* (112) expressed it: "an eye for an eye and a tooth for a tooth."

An understanding of the origin and purpose of this impulse helps to explain why its mastery is so important. The small child, particularly the borderline child because of the deprivation he experiences, feels helpless to protect himself against emotional suffering and stores the pain, which brings with it a resolve (a) never to permit this passive acceptance of pain again and (b) to pay back the real and/or imagined perpetrators of this and other pain when he gets big enough. The impulse is to overcome the

182

childhood trauma by replaying the past in the present, only this time with the opposite result. Instead of being weak, small, helpless, a passive object, the individual is strong, active and meting out just punishment for the trauma and thereby undoing the past. The talionic impulse seeks immediate release without regard to consequences, particularly its effect on future or long-term objectives.

The Talionic Impulse and Society

An understanding of the social origins of the talionic impulse gives added perspective. The concept of an objective sense of the rightness or wrongness of human conduct is a relative newcomer in the evolution of civilization and is the product of a long, slow process of change. It did not spring full-grown like Athena from the head of Zeus. Its evolution reflects the struggle at a social level to internalize what Nietzsche (91) called the cruelty streak.

This impulse in the individual has been socialized, ritualized, and institutionalized over the centuries (20, 91). The behavioral excesses that flowed from this impulse were rife in the Middle Ages: "to behold suffering gave pleasure, but to cause another to suffer afforded an even greater pleasure . . . a royal wedding or great public celebration would have been incomplete without executions, tortures, or autos-da-fé . . . there was scarcely a noble household without some person whose office it was to serve as a butt for everyone's malice and cruel teasing" (91). It was literally incorporated into the legal system: "The creditor had the right to inflict all manner of indignity and pain on the body of the defaulting debtor. For example, he could cut out an amount of flesh proportionate to the amount of the debt, and we find, very early, quite detailed legal assessments of the value of individual parts of the body. An equivalence is provided by the creditor's receiving, in place of material compensation such as money, land, or other possessions, a kind of pleasure. That pleasure is induced by his being able to exercise his power freely upon one who is powerless" (91).

Nietzsche (91) despaired, as we often do today, of the talionic urge ever being completely mastered by the individual: "Should it actually come to pass that the just man remains just even toward his despoiler (and not simply cool, moderate, distant, indifferent) to be just is a positive attitude, and that even under the stress of hurt, contumely, denigration, the noble, penetrating yet mild objectivity of the just (the judging) eye does not become clouded, then we have before us an instance of the rarest accomplishment, something that, if we are wise, we will neither expect nor be too easily convinced of. It is generally true of even the most decent people that a small dose of insult, malice, insinuation is enough to send the blood to their eyes and equity out the window."

One cannot read Tuchman's (113) history of the Middle Ages without marveling at the lusty joy of the knights as they hacked each other to pieces, or at the remarkable propensity of the common people—the usual victims—to take pleasure in overt acts of cruelty such as murder, rape, crucifixion, pillage and maiming. If one considers for a moment how commonly the children in those days were exposed in early childhood to extreme deprivations, it explains, as I shall elaborate later, one of the motives for such behavior.

These sanctioned social spectacles disappeared as civilization developed. The propensity to act out the talionic impulse had been internalized. Nietzsche (91) stated: "The formidable bulwarks by means of which the polity protected itself against the ancient instincts of freedom (punishment was one of the strongest of these bulwarks) caused those wild, extravagant instincts to turn in upon man. Hostility, cruelty, the delight in persecution, raids, excitement, destruction, all turned against their begetter. Lacking external enemies and resistances, and confined within an oppressive narrowness and regularity, man began rending, persecuting, terrifying himself, like a wild beast hurling itself against the bars of its cage."

Freud (20) phrased it as follows: "His aggressiveness was introjected, internalized; it was, in point of fact, sent back to where it came from—that is, it was directed towards his own ego. There it was taken over by a portion of the ego, which set itself over against the rest of the ego as superego, and which now, in the form of "conscience," was ready to put into action against the ego the same harsh aggressiveness that the ego would have liked to satisfy upon other, extraneous individuals." Along with this development came the increased influence of conscience, guilt, duty, laws, religion and morality.

TALIONIC IMPULSE AND THE INDIVIDUAL

Ontogeny follows phylogeny in emotional development as well as in physical development. The individual repeats in his development the same stages and struggles the civilization went through. A person's objective sense of the rightness or wrongness of human conduct is an achievement, an end product of a long, slow, tedious process which requires the mastery of separation anxiety, along with the internalization and mastery of the talionic impulse, followed by the overcoming of castration anxiety and the incest taboo with its rigid and extensive defensive prohibitions against instinct (27).

Only after the talionic impulse has been subdued and mastered and the rigid and global extensions of the incest taboo prohibitions overcome can the superego become emancipated during adolescence from its dependence on the introjected images of the parents. This frees the psychic structure to weigh objective realities and take them in to design a unique personal morality. In the course of this development, the intrapsychic structure evolves through stages into whole self and object representations with an autonomous, effectively functioning ego that allows the person to perceive reality clearly, contain the uncomfortable affects a moral dilemma may raise, and use reason as a means of coping or adaptation. The apex of personality development is to have the capacity to take full responsibility for the self, its wishes, its acts, and their consequences. The length and complexity of this developmental pathway underscore its vulnerability to detours and arrests along the way, all of which affect the end product, i.e., the individual's objective sense of the rightness or wrongness of human conduct.

This process is facilitated and eased by appropriate parenting, which minimizes and repairs the inevitable developmental traumata. Since there is not so much hurt and suffering, there is less talionic impulse and less need for vengeance. The talionic impulse is, for the most part, overcome, and aggression is freed to find release in self-assertive efforts at mastery and adaptation.

VICISSITUDES OF THE TALIONIC IMPULSE IN THE BORDERLINE PATIENT

To begin with a clinical example: When one hears of the adolescent gang that poured gasoline over an old derelict, set him afire and laughed as he burned, one's sense of human morality is shocked. This shock is compounded when one learns that these adolescents had no remorse or guilt feelings. They felt and treated the derelict like an inanimate object who provided an opportunity for them to feel pleasure by inflicting pain—shades of the Middle Ages!

A second example: the sexual sadist who writes messages on the mirror with lipstick for someone to restrain him but continues to sexually abuse and murder.

In many instances, this "wrong" conduct is motivated by the talionic impulse—an eye for an eye and a tooth for a tooth. When one examines the past histories of these individuals, one finds evidence of such cruel, barbarous, torturous exploitation of their infantile dependence and helplessness that even their later-life crimes, heinous as they are, pale by comparison. They seem to be carrying out that deepest and most ancient of human responses, the talionic impulse—an automatic defensive response to inflict injury when injured.

Who is responsible here for what? Do we blame the original infantile situation that planted the bomb or the later adult who exploded it? The adult cannot use his past as an excuse to avoid responsibility for his actions in the present (though how many patients do we hear doing this very thing?), but it is highly un-likely, in these cases, that the present would have occurred with-out the past conditioning. It is all too easy to relieve oneself of having to deal with the ambiguities and complexities of this chicken and egg dilemma by retreating to a horrified condemna-tion of the act. Let us take it a step further. Since the parents who carried out the torture were also compelled to exact talionic retri-bution, are they more responsible? Perhaps we could say society's institutions are responsible for failing to identify and treat the parents before they could torture the child who later killed the old man. This reductio ad absurdum argument leads to the fol-lowing conclusion: Terrible tragedies are inflicted on many children during their early developmental years which plant time bombs that go off later in life. Even though the child had no con-trol over the planting of the bomb, when he grows up, he has to take responsibility for its effects.

The psychoanalytic study of the arrested structures of the bor-derline patient provides a window on early developmental proc-esses in the individual that is analogous to the window provided on ancient civilizations by the ruins of Pompeii, which was ar-rested and fixed in 79 A.D., by the explosion of Mt. Vesuvius. At Pompeii, we can study the forerunners of many aspects of current civilization, i.e., religion, culture, art, entertainment. In the bor-derline patient, we can study in bold relief some of the precursors in development of the intra-psychic structures that will later evolve into a sense of morality.

In the borderline patient (83, 86, 96), there is a gross miscar-riage of the early developmental process which results in a kind of throwback for the individual to an earlier stage of civilization where the talionic impulse was acted out. However, in these cases, the talionic impulse is internalized and acted out not on others but on the self—a caricature of Freud's (20) and Nietzsche's (91) views of how civilization developed.

The borderline child (86) experiences the parents' exploitation of his dependency and helplessness as the grossest form of cruelty and torture. This leads to an abandonment depression, an essential part of which is rage. Unable to express his hurt and rage because of his need for and fear of his parents, he attempts to master it by internalizing it, using the mechanism of identification with the aggressor. He creates an internalized drama of a medieval spectacle, where the patient is both attacker and victim. He discharges the rage by attacking himself, fantasying revenge on the parents and fulfillment of his talionic impulses by destroying their possession. This is at the same time a defense against the underlying talionic, homicidal urges toward the exploiting object. There is also a compensatory accompanying fantasy that, if he dramatizes his sorrowful state sufficiently, the parents will provide the wished-for response. This results in a failure to master the talionic impulse, which is destructively acted out on the self. Aggression is thus not free for release in self-assertive, adaptive behavior.

This dynamic has lain at the core of the symptomatology of every borderline patient I have treated. He wants primarily revenge, to get back—not to get better. The second critical crossroad comes in treatment when the patient must make a choice between getting back or getting better. He cannot have both. As long as his aggression is channeled into revenge, it is not available to build psychic structure. He must give up the idea of revenge, that is, he must master the talionic impulse, and free his aggression to be used to support his self-image, rather than to attack it. By overcoming and mastering his talionic urge for revenge, he lays the groundwork for the beginning of an objective sense of morality—he puts aside the immediate but destructive and fantasy pleasure of revenge for the more long-term but more realistic objective and enduring satisfaction of aiding and abetting his own growth. He tolerates current discomfort in pursuit of future objectives.

What happens, you may well ask, to that rageful urge for revenge? Part is discharged in interviews and part is sublimated and discharged through active support of various social causes and groups that come to have a personal meaning—the poor, the deprived, the handicapped, those being treated unfairly or unjustly by authorities or society. Sometimes these are combined and channeled into a career identity—the reporter who investigates the corruption of politicians, the lawyer who defends the poor and the powerless, the labor leader who battles the capitalists, the writer who exposes the evils of society.

Two case presentations—Fred, who has been presented earlier, and Paul—illustrate the vicissitudes of the talionic impulse in the borderline patient in treatment.

CASE ILLUSTRATIONS

Fred F.

Fred's early developmental deprivations resulted in the following dynamic: If Fred gave up his individuality, his self, his own thoughts, feelings and assertiveness, and submitted passively, the father would love him and take care of him. Initiative, activity, self-assertion and anger must be inhibited, along with all associated activies such as learning, or they would induce the father's withdrawal of approval. However, this idea of approval for submission derived from fantasies Fred elaborated from the father's verbalizations of love for him—verbalizations which were empty of substance, as in reality the father neglected Fred.

As Fred began psychotherapy, this theme was reproduced in the transference. His inhibitions produced great difficulty in talking and associating, and he expected me to resonate with the second part of the dynamic; that is, I should take over for him like a father and direct him. When I did not, but confronted him with his behavior, the underlying talionic rage at my not taking care of him (like a father) burst forth, not verbally, but in all kinds of resistant behavior—missing interviews, being late for interviews, blocking, etc. Fred expressed it in typical fashion by actions destructive to himself. When the resistance was dealt with by confrontation, Fred became aware of the self-destructive nature of his behavior, controlled it and began to investigate the underlying psychodynamics: what he called his lifelong search for a father that "had prevented me from getting involved in doing my own thing; my self wants to come out, but my need for a father overrides it."

As Fred ventilated and explored his depression and anger, the inhibitions lifted and he resumed school. However, at crucial points, as he again and again came to the point of facing his feelings of hopelessness and his homicidal talionic rage about the father, his need to defend would produce severe blocking in sessions and the learning inhibition would return.

When I pointed out the relationship between these two, Fred exploded with: "I don't want to get better, I don't want to do it myself. I want a father. I want to get what I was deprived of in childhood." When I underlined the conflict between this defensive wish and his own growth, Fred responded: "I felt a responsibility to my father not to be angry, so I had to put the anger on myself. If I make myself hopeless enough, he will have to take care of me. I am killing myself to keep from killing my father." As Fred worked through this talionic rage, he began to master it, which freed his aggression to support his self-assertive attempts to adapt to reality.

A key shift in momentum had taken place in the treatment from the acting-out of revenge to the control of these impulses in the service of growth. Concomitantly, Fred's intellectual powers were freed to attend to the task of learning, and he eventually completed treatment and graduated college with honors. His objective had been to become an architect. The aggression was freed not only to become invested in the act of learning but eventually to be sublimated and expressed through his identity as an architect who works as a city planner to better the welfare of the poor.

Paul H.

Paul, age 23, had a long history, beginning in high school, of depression, passive-aggressive acting-out and obsessive thinking. He had barely managed to get through high school, and it took him six years to complete college because of his avoidance, passive-aggressive acting-out and drug ingestion. He saw a therapist from once to three times a week all six years of college. When he finally graduated, his depression mounted, he couldn't function, so he returned home to live and came to me for treatment, furious at his therapist that he wasn't any better.

Paul's brother, who had minimal brain disorder, was the mother's favorite. The mother, fearing that Paul would outshine the brother, attacked all of Paul's efforts at individuation while indulging his avoidance and passivity and inappropriately sexually stimulating him. The father, on the other hand, apparently showed a narcissistic disorder. He required that Paul sacrifice his individuation in order to provide a mirroring object for the father. The father seemed to take delight in exposing Paul to humiliation.

The resulting dynamics was similar to Fred's. Paul reproduced in the transference the interaction with his father. He would attack his own assertive coping efforts, retreat into depression and passivity and expect me to take over for him, as his previous therapist had no doubt done. When, rather than take over for him, I confronted Paul with this behavior, he expressed his talionic rage (not like Fred by blocking or missing interviews) by giving up any attempt at therapeutic investigation and plunging into passive reveries that revolved around fantasies either of being taken care of or of his own grandiosity. Paul was acting out his talionic rage on himself in the transference to get revenge on me (them) and coerce me (them) to take care of him.

Paul also was a very talented pianist but had been blocked by the need to express aggression against himself. When piano practice was going well, he would respond as he did in interviews. He would block out all feeling, give up practice (individuation) and retreat into defensive reveries. Extensive confrontation of the destructiveness of this behavior led Paul to control it and to investigate the underlying abandonment depression with its talionic rage. He reported: "I had to be miserable to get my parents' attention. I have to be in a state of intolerable suffering, helpless, powerless, abandoned, to please them. The evil of it is staggering."

Paul framed his childhood memories in World War II prison-camp metaphors with himself as the helpless prisoner and his parents as the brutal German guards. He envisioned only two options for himself: to be passive, the tortured prisoner, or to assert himself and become the brutal guard, which would make his parents the tortured inmates. There was no way out.

In therapy his talionic rage gradually emerged: "I'd get violently angry and want to strike out physically at them, kick their heads in, kill them. This frightened me. I would be without them." He then suddenly reported: "I just had this terrifying realization. I am possessed by a passion to torture myself to hurt them, to get back at them. If they saw me in a horrible-enough condition, it would pay them back. But it does no good. It's hopeless. They don't care."

Paul's fantasies of talionic revenge were gradually ventilated and worked through. His aggression was freed to find release in self-assertive adaptation. He became able to practice the piano freely, and his skill improved dramatically. His obsessive preoccupation with prison-camp metaphors diminished and was replaced by a new and absorbing interest in his own self-assertion. As his debut as a concert pianist approached, he suddenly informed me emphatically that he would start his career as an"orthodox Jew, yarmulke and all." I asked why. He replied defiantly: "The Nazis had their games, now we'll see."

Paul had mastered his talionic impulse and made an adaptive sublimation of his aggression which was accompanied by a dramatic, constructive transformation of his self-image into a self-assertive concert pianist. The freeing of his aggression enabled him to shift his identification.

Summary

Psychotherapeutic work with patients with developmental arrests provides a unique window from which to observe and study the early emotional struggles that precede and are a prelude to the formation of mature intrapsychic structures, which themselves form the basis for such mature human capacities as a sense of morality.

An analogy is drawn between the role of the mastery of the talionic impulse in the development of morality in civilization and in the development of morality in the individual. Two clinical illustrations were presented which describe how the talionic impulse which was acted out against the self is mastered and the underlying aggression is freed to find release in constructive, self-assertive efforts at coping and adaptation.

A theory is presented that a true sense of morality cannot be achieved until the talionic impulse is mastered. The acute stage of this battle takes place early in development, the first three years, and success leads to the second important struggle—the resolution of castration anxiety. Successful mastery of these two developmental struggles forms two of the essential roots of an adult sense of morality.

The other patients presented in this volume show the same theme. Ann expressed her rage through somatic symptoms. Her resultant helplessness coerced the environment into fulfilling her fantasy of being taken care of. Leslie's resort to extremely elaborate and revengeful sexual fantasies threatened to defeat her treatment.

The first critical turning point of treatment, which results in the consolidation of the therapeutic alliance, is the patient's recognition of the alien quality of the defenses of his pathologic ego. The second critical turning point is the patient's recognition of the vengeful and utterly self-destructive nature of his talionic needs, followed by the decision to give up revenge in order to get better.

12

Termination
of Treatment

Although there are many articles in the literature on termination of treatment (17), few refer to the borderline patient, whose difficulties with separation make handling of termination crucial, since it tests how much treatment has improved the patient's ability to manage separation stress.

The awesome power of mankind's dependency needs is illustrated by the prolonged state of physical and, therefore, emotional dependence of man's early development, which contrasts markedly with that period of life in animals. This difference is believed by evolutionary theorists to have evolved over time in order to prepare man for a life so much more complex than that of animals. Mahler (74) emphasized the profound emotional effects of this prolonged period of dependence in saying "man's lifelong, albeit decreasing, dependence."

The dependency needs are one of the vehicles not only for biologic development but also for psychological development of the human being—as the child learns to sit up, talk and walk, his psyche also grows. When the dependency needs are handled appropriately, they become building blocks for personality structure; when handled inappropriately, they make major contributions to psychopathology.

The power of the abuse of dependency needs can be seen in hospitalized borderline adolescents who showed difficulty in giving up the dependency gratifications of the hospital environment when it came time for them to leave the hospital and begin to function on their own (86, 87). As a consultant to a halfway house for the most disturbed black delinquent teenagers in New York City, I observed time and again these teenagers reporting, on the one hand, that their mothers had tried to kill them by putting their head in the oven or by stabbing them; on the other hand, they would all verbalize that their dearest wish was to leave the halfway house and return home to that mother. In a study of the treatment termination of patients in psychoanalysis, almost all expressed the wish that the treatment could go on forever.

The dependency needs of borderline patients were severely frustrated and traumatized in their early development, and one of the goals of treatment has been the attenuation and repair of the effects of that trauma (83). Termination becomes crucial because it tests the degree to which that attenuation and repair have taken place--the degree to which the patient can be independent and take responsibility for and be able to manage himself in a constructive, adaptive manner. In more technical terms, it tests the degree to which the patients have internalized the object and repaired their ego defects so that their intrapsychic structure is now strong enough to enable them to manage for themselves.

In our follow-up of improved borderline adolescents (87), we were able to demonstrate that, in treatment, the patient gradually decreases his libidinal investment of the object and increases his libidinal investment of the self and that this movement or change is accompanied by and associated with slow, gradual, improved functioning and diminishing of symptoms. However, the greatest improvement comes about only from full separation of the self-representation from the object representation, which brings with it the greatest strengthening of the ego and the liberation of the capacities for autonomy, intimacy and creativity.

All patients cannot achieve this optimum goal of separation of the self-representation from the object representation. Some, regardless of therapeutic input, do not seem able to adequately internalize the object and they, therefore, represent very poor therapeutic risks. Those who cannot, however, are entitled to a trial of treatment to see how far along the continuum of internalization they can come.

TERMINATION OF UNSUCCESSFUL TREATMENT

Many factors can result in the termination of unsuccessful treatment of borderline patients. Some borderline patients are not motivated to participate in therapy unless they can find some way to manipulate the therapist into resonating with their rewarding object relations part-unit or "taking care of them." They will stay with the therapist who responds for many years, achieving fantasy gratification at the cost of therapeutic progress. However, as soon as the therapist sets limits to these regressive manipulations, the patient is no longer interested in treatment and will stop. This can sometimes come about as early as during the evaluation if the patient perceives that the therapist will not respond to his manipulations.

In my work with patients, my concern as to whether or not they will continue treatment has always been subordinated to my concern as to whether or not I had done an appropriate job. If I had, my mind was at ease, realizing that I had no more control over whether the patient stayed in treatment or stopped. In addition, I have yet to hear of a patient who left treatment because I did not resonate with the rewarding unit and then continued successfully with another therapist.

A particularly dramatic example was an artist in the mid-thirties with drug addiction and severe sexual problems who had

had several unsuccessful trials of treatment with other therapists. He had manipulated his girlfriend into managing his life, as well as into paying for his treatment. When she reneged on payment and I insisted that the bill be paid, i.e., when he had to take responsibility for himself and pay, he abruptly stopped treatment.

Some patients with a distancing transference have such an intense fear of being abandoned by the therapist that early in treatment they may react to separation stress, such as the therapist's becoming ill or going on vacation, by acting out through stopping treatment. Others, after their initial problems in adaptation and coping are cleared up, become frightened at becoming more involved in treatment because it heightens their fears of engulfment or abandonment and they defend by a flight into "health" and stop treatment.

A common experience is the borderline patient who, as he becomes more involved in treatment, finds a relationship outside the therapy—either a heterosexual or homosexual one—which he uses as a hedge against the transference relationship. He titrates that relationship against the transference—when involvement in the transference increases anxiety, he decreases the treatment and increases involvement in the relationship. Some of these patients eventually marry the partner in order to avoid working through the depression in therapy.

Finally, there are some adolescents who are so mired in the distorted communications and role conflicts with their parents that they cannot allow themselves to participate in treatment until they receive permission from the parent.

A 16-year-old girl with serious school failure denied and avoided any meaningful emotional content in initial sessions. Both father and mother had successful careers and spent all their time at work; during the little time that was spent at home, the entire family catered to and was ruled by the narcissistic needs of the father, who could not be challenged. Joint interviews where the therapist brought this to the family's attention had an immediate and dramatic result in the adolescent patient's individual sessions where, having been given indirect permission through the joint session, she dropped the denial and avoidance and immediately began to talk about the conflicts at home. However, a number of months later, when her parents stopped their sessions, the adolescent patient returned to denial and avoidance.

SUCCESSFUL TERMINATION

Confrontive or Supportive Psychotherapy

The goal of confrontive psychotherapy (called in previous publications supportive), more limited than that of intensive psychoanalytic psychotherapy, is improvement to the point that adaptation is no longer sacrificed to defense. The projections of the wish-for-reunion fantasies upon the environment and reality are removed, reality perception improves along with the patient's capacity to assert himself, so that he perceives and copes with reality in an appropriate and adaptive manner as much as possible in his best interest, resorting very little to regressive, destructive behavior.

At termination the patient should have found more sublimative, adaptive modes for containing his depression. His functioning at work, in relationships and in the pursuit of his interests should be more consistent and active, with more personal satisfaction.

He does not achieve the flowering of individuation with the increase in capacity for intimacy, autonomy and creativity. The vulnerability to separation stress remains, although it is somewhat less intense and better defended against by a stronger ego. The chief remaining problem is his difficulties in object relations due to remaining fears of engulfment and/or abandonment, which the patient must learn to contain.

Some patients may have to be seen once or twice a week for the rest of their lives. I see no objection to this, with the proviso that the therapist does not resonate with the rewarding unit and collude in a regressive experience but continues to confront, and the patient consequently continues to show changes in adaptation.

Developmental time and the time perception of real life differ. Some borderline patients have been so heavily traumatized in early development that they cannot maintain a barely adequate level of adaptation without therapeutic support. In others the degree of early trauma is such that the patient improves at a snail's pace. Most medical treatment does not offer cure but improvement, and many medical patients are on maintenance therapy their entire lives. Why should we expect psychiatry to be any different? On the other hand, this perspective must be carefully carried out, evaluating each individual patient in the context of his early developmental traumas and potentials and not in terms of any rigid, idealistic goals of the therapist. It should not be used as an argument by the therapist to collude with a patient's resistance and to avoid growth and change.

Intensive Psychoanalytic Psychotherapy

The goals of intensive psychoanalytic psychotherapy, more ambitious than confrontive therapy, are the following: Symptoms markedly attenuated, functioning markedly improved, with little or no sacrifice of adaptation to defense. The split part-units have consolidated to form whole-units as the patient achieves the stage of on-the-way-to-object constancy or whole object relations. He perceives objects as wholes, both good and bad, and his investment in the object can persist despite frustration. He is able to evoke the image of the object when it is not present. The ego defects have been substantially repaired, with an improvement in reality perception, particularly about self-object representations and parental figures, i.e., the ability to see parents as they are and not through infantile fantasies.

There should be parallel maturation of ego structure and defenses, with splitting becoming supplanted by repression, reaction formation and sublimation, with the disappearance of clinging, acting-out and avoidance. Ego structure should improve, with a strengthening of ego functions, reality perception, frustration tolerance, impulse control and ego boundaries.

The patient should be able to activate himself to implement his interests and wishes in reality through self-assertive behavior, without avoidance of an individuative stimulus. He should be able to autonomously regulate his self-esteem, with flexibility to negotiate a variety of possible solutions to tensions between id, superego and reality. There should be a resultant flowering of individuation, with an increase in the capacities for creativity, intimacy and independence.

This obviously is an ideal and individual patients will make relative degrees of progress toward this goal, depending upon the severity of their disorder and their capacity for treatment, as well as the therapist's skill. If the disorder is not too severe, if the patient has a good capacity for treatment and a good therapist and life treats him with kindness, the ultimate goal may be achieved. Some severely ill patients, however, can be said to have had a successful therapy even if they are far from this model. For example, if analysis enables a nonfunctional patient to function, even at an isolated level, one far below that which would be optimum for most healthy people, it would still seem an adequate achievement for this patient with his background.

The Clinical Picture of Termination

The borderline patient's principal intrapsychic problem has been the inability to fully separate from the mother object representation and develop to the stage of on-the-way-to-object-constancy—in other words, to manage himself autonomously on his own. Therefore, termination itself has some features specific to the borderline, in that it tests the adequacy of the whole therapeutic process. Previous phases of the treatment which had been aborted or not adequately worked through will return to haunt the termination process. Despite the prior difficulties experienced in treatment, this termination phase is probably, technically speaking, the most difficult.

The patient now feels well and is functioning well for the most part. Resistances and defenses are harder to work with, as the therapist has less leverage. The patient can point to his indisputably better adjustment to back up his claim that this is not a resistance to termination but actually an act of termination itself. The therapist in this situation has little to rely upon except his opinion and the strength of transference.

The patient has progressed to this point in treatment on the basis of a fantasy acted out in the transference of exclusive possession of his therapist, representing the patient's wish for exclusive possession of the mother—the mother who will always be wished for—to provide support for separation-individuation. Within this transference fantasy, he has worked through his abandonment depression, separated from the object representation of the mother, and his ego has grown.

Now he must turn in this last dramatic phase of therapy to work through this fantasy of exclusive possession of his therapist in order to develop fully to the stage of on-the-way-to object constancy. This stress automatically triggers all prior separation reactions that have been worked through and flushes out some that were overlooked or avoided.

A second theme that emerges as the termination approaches takes on added weight: the patient's anxiety about having to function on his own. As this occurs, the patient then activates his old defenses against abandonment depression, and these must be worked through. Ordinarily, new themes do not arise but old ones are reexacerbated with old defenses in the transference, either clinging or distancing. However, new historical information and links may emerge. The therapist must be on guard against various forms of acting-out whose purpose is to abort the evolution of this final mourning process.

No new therapeutic techniques are necessary at this phase but mainly continuing application of the old techniques. Ordinarily the suggestion for termination should come from the patient, who then has to be given time and opportunity to work it through. In some cases, a weaning schedule might be best; in others not. The therapist's availability after termination should be assumed and not expressed or elaborated upon. The therapist does not alter his therapeutically objective role at the time of termination. This is no time for "becoming friends" with the patient or indulging in fantasies of future contacts; these would all interfere with the extensive working-through process which continues after the last contact with the therapist.

Countertransference problems to termination are perhaps the most common, the most intense and the most denied of all countertransference problems. In early unsuccessful terminations, there can be anxiety and guilt about having used inappropriate therapeutic techniques or having been provoked to express one's annoyance or anger with a patient, thereby causing the patient to leave, or feelings of inadequacy as a therapist that patients leave. Sometimes there are clinging reactions to the patient's leaving in order to preserve one's image as an effective therapist. Sometimes, unfortunately, practical reasons enter the matter, for the therapist who does not have enough patients may overlook the ancient rule that one's therapeutic actions should put the patient's interests and not the therapist's first.

In patients who are successfully treated with intensive psychoanalytic psychotherapy, an emotional harmony of interaction evolves between therapist and patient which is intensely gratifying to the therapist as well as to the patient. It resembles but is obviously not the same as the earlier intense symbiotic interactions with the mother. The therapist's rescue fantasies and his fantasies of omnipotence become reinforced in the daily toil, as the intricacies of the patient's dynamics gradually unfold, mysteries yield to the light of reason and the patient improves. It is often as difficult for the therapist to give up this gratification provided by his patient as it is for the patient to give up his fantasies of exclusive possession of the therapist as a maternal part-object. Sometimes it is more difficult.

The bare bones of this issue were dramatically revealed in our inpatient service where the therapist had complete control of the patient and his life, therefore serving in addition as a parental surrogate. This fact further enhanced the therapist's rescue and omnipotent fantasies; at discharge he had to turn all of these controls back to the patient. It became an axiom that everybody on the unit—nurses, occupational and recreational therapists, supervisors and even the other patients—was fully aware of the patient's readiness for discharge before the therapist was. Dramatic confrontations and arguments developed between supervisor and resident therapist over this issue, and on rare occasions, the resident had to be ordered to discharge the patient when the issue could not be resolved through discussion.

Occasionally, therapists respond to their anxiety about termination by clinging responses revealed in various measures such as weaning rather than stopping, prolonged telephone contacts or attempting to shift roles from that of a therapist to some version of a "friend."

One often wonders how many of the instances where therapists marry their patients spring from the therapists' anxiety about termination. The patient has progressed in treatment to the termination phase. Therapist and patient can figure out no other way to continue the relationship without formalizing it through the institution of marriage.

Therapists can entertain all sorts of fantasies of various levels of participation in the patient's posttreatment real life, including actual physical interaction through friendship, participation in some of the patient's activities or some form of regular or irregular reporting, etc. Reflecting on the observations of patients terminating psychoanalysis, that all patients studied had a wish for the transference to continue forever, gives an idea of the harmful effect it would have on the patient if these fantasies were acted out. Perhaps an occasional report by letter or postcard does not have to be detrimental if it is prompted by the patient—not by the therapist.

Therapists can also have more serious psychopathology that affects termination. The borderline therapist with clinging defenses will probably not observe that his patient is ready for termination, will retard the patient's development and activate his own clinging responses. On the other hand, the therapist with the distancing defenses may prematurely terminate the treatment before the patient has an opportunity to get involved. I recall a therapist telling me that he had no problems with termination because when that phase of treatment arose he had a nurse-therapist to whom he referred all his patients to deal with termination.

One can only speculate on the kinds of problems this presents in various analytic institutes where the patient, once terminated, then has a more or less close, professional and perhaps even personal contact with his former therapist. While there is some question as to the amount of emotional damage therapists with neuroses might suffer from by this arrangement, it seems pretty clear that borderline therapists in this sort of situation are bound to have their final working-through process impaired. This certainly could lead to the development of cults around individual therapists who could not let their analysands go, and the relationship could be acted out in various kinds of intellectual or theoretical conflicts within institutes.

These problems make abundantly clear the reasons for my earlier comments about the therapeutic frame and why it is necessary to maintain therapeutic objectivity and neutrality, i.e., to present to the patient a clear model of the therapist's ability to perceive the difference between the self-representation and the object representation and to maintain the limits of this perception. This not only presents a role model for the patient to learn and protects the therapeutic framework against the patient's acting-out but also prepares from the opening gun the bedrock for eventual termination, i.e., we are two separate people getting together on a temporary basis to perform a task which, when completed, will end the reason for our being together.

ACTING-OUT AS A FORM OF TERMINATION

Acting-out as a form of termination can occur at any time, in any phase of the treatment for a variety of reasons, for example in response to therapeutic errors, to intercurrent events in the patient's life as well as to vicissitudes within the therapy itself. We are concerned here principally with two points in the treatment which are particularly vulnerable to a termination by acting-out. First, it may occur in a patient in confrontive therapy, after the initial maladaptive behavior has been contained. The patient is no longer sacrificing adaptation to defense, his life structure has improved markedly, but he is feeling more depression. He must move either further into an analytic form of treatment to work through the abandonment depression or find some other means of defending against it.

At this point the patient will often act out either through a marriage or a relationship or through moving away as a means of defending against further involvement with the therapist and his abandonment depression. It is particularly difficult because the usual therapeutic leverage of the patient's symptomatic difficulty in functioning is gone; in addition, the patient is often able to minimize and deny his problems in relationships as well as the variations in his affective state. He may well argue that the level of his adaptation is proof enough that he no longer needs treatment and that the therapist is trying to hold on to him.

The future course of patients who terminate in this fashion usually consists of more or less continued adaptive behavior barring separation stress—in other words, pretty good functioning but difficulty with object relations and with the episodic appearance of symptoms.

The second point occurs with the patient in intensive psychoanalytic psychotherapy who has, over a period of years, worked through the abandonment depression and is in the last or separation phase of treatment and, rather than stick it out and work through the separation of the intrapsychic object representation of the therapist from the self-representation, the patient defends against this separation anxiety by stopping treatment or terminating. He thereby gains the illusion of autonomy or independence, while he is still not fully separated from the intrapsychic object representation of the therapist.

The question is often raised as to what is wrong with this result. What more can be expected? The answer is that the patient of course is doing a great deal better, but that he still remains to a certain degree dependent upon that object and, therefore, does not have full autonomy of his ego, nor has he developed to full, whole-object relations, since he must retain various fantasies about his therapist and, therefore, cannot see him in reality as he is. This will then have subtle but definite influence on his eventual capacity for intimacy or autonomy and creativity, as well as on his object relations. This type of termination by acting-out is even more difficult for the therapist to deal with than the one mentioned above, since the patient's overall adaptation and his object relations are indeed markedly improved and his symptomatic state greatly attenuated. The therapist's point of view can often be seen by the patient as being rather abstract, academic and perfectionistic and having little to do with him. Both of these types of termination by acting-out are illustrated below.

Case Illustration

Confrontive Therapy—Catherine

The treatment of the first patient, Catherine, was previously reported (83), and the reader is referred to that report for the details. In brief, Catherine, 22, came to treatment complaining of depression, loneliness, inability to commit herself to a career or a relationship and a long history of defending herself against abandonment depression by sexual acting-out in relationships. After four years of treatment, she had progressed to the point where her fear of engulfment had so lessened that she was able to find a seemingly appropriate male partner. He seemed to fall in love with her, and after a six-month period of experimentation, they decided to marry. At this point, she decided to stop treatment and to continue the work on her own.

Although she had made remarkable improvement over the four years, to the point that her life structure was no longer destructive and she seemed able to manage her fear of engulfment enough to form a relationship, the fact that the termination was by acting-out did not become clear until she returned two years later.

After stopping treatment, her relationship with her husband had been fine, as she worked as a teacher and he at his job. They had their apartment, and he shared the chores. He was "overly generous," required very little of her and constantly pushed money on her to buy things for herself. On the other hand, she found him to be rather rigid and authoritarian, with very little insight into his own feelings and even less capacity to respond empathetically to hers. She felt she had more or less traded off the satisfactions of his generous treatment of her for the emotional frustrations of his limited capacity for relating to her.

This precarious balance was maintained for about 18 months, until she broached the subject of having a baby and moving to a house in the suburbs. He responded that he was not interested, as he already had one baby in the family and did not want two. She reacted with depression and fury and withdrew.

Shortly thereafter she met a fellow teacher who was everything her husband was not: responsive, emotional, in touch with his own feelings. She began an affair with him.

It became clear from this story that she had stopped treatment to act out a defense against taking full responsibility for herself and facing in the sessions the intrapsychic withdrawing object representation of the father, which had remained split from the rewarding-unit representation. Rather than face this, she stopped treatment and acted out through finding a man who would resonate with the rewarding unit, and she, therefore, could carry out the fantasy of being a little girl with a father who loved her. Her husband infantilized her as a substitute for emotional relating, and she accepted it.

This tenuous compromise, however, fell apart, when she now wished to have a baby, despite the fact that she had allowed her husband to treat her as a baby. She saw no inconsistency in this, and when he now frustrated her wishes, he no longer resonated with the rewarding unit, triggering her rage. She projected the withdrawing unit on him and, in keeping with her splitting defense, started an affair with a man who now became the rewarding unit, the original split with the father now being reestablished between the husband (the withdrawing unit) and the lover (the rewarding unit).

This second level of defense was then interrupted by the lover confronting her that she would either have to give up the husband or stop the affair, that he really was in love with her and wanted her to be with him. This, of course, would have required her to take responsibility for herself and for her own wishes, as well as require her to overcome the splitting defense. She felt paralyzed, unable to move and in that setting came to see me.

In a series of consultation interviews, I, on the one hand, empathized with the environmental and intrapsychic difficulties presented in the conflict with her husband and in the affair, but, on the other hand, suggested that the motivation for the consultation was the same as for the affair: that since her husband had not taken care of her by offering to provide a baby in addition to all the other rewards, she had in disappointment and despair turned from him to the lover; and since the lover was now not going to take responsibility for her and provide for her welfare, she was turning to me and expecting me to do it.

The basic problem was that, when she had come in treatment to face the need to be responsible for herself, to give up the fantasy of a father who would love her and take care of her, and to face her anger and depression, she had instead found a suitable person to act out the fantasy and stopped treatment. This fantasy had in it the seeds of its own frustration and destruction. My advice was for her to again try to deal with it in treatment.

In essence, the problem was neither the husband nor the lover but herself and her unwillingness to take responsibility for herself, which was crucially relevant to her present environmental situation. If she made any decision, she would have to pay the consequences, but she still felt herself unable to decide. At the same time, I cautioned her that if she did not make a conscious decision regarding the affair and deal with the consequences, there was a possibility that life events, i.e., discovery of the affair, would make the decision for her and present more consequences to deal with. Within a very short time, it became clear that she really had no more motivation to work on the problem now than she had had when she left treatment, that she really did not want to do anything about giving up this fantasy and becoming responsible for herself. I pointed out to her that to continue treatment knowing that sort of motivation would be to collude with it, and I thought it would be better if she stopped until she could make some decision. After several interviews she agreed to stop, saying that she thought she would end the affair, since she really didn't want to make any decision regarding treatment, i.e., working to become independent. I have not heard from her since.

Separation Phase of Intensive Psychoanalytic Psychotherapy

The first two cases below are of adolescents who had intensive psychoanalytic psychotherapy over a number of years, received substantial benefit and then terminated by acting-out at the point when they would have had to work through their separation from the intrapsychic image of the therapist in the last phases of therapy.

Both of these patients have been described in detail in another volume (87), so they will only briefly be summarized here, along with some observations on the ten-year follow-up.

Case Illustrations

Joe S.

The first patient, Joe, was seen at the age of 16 for severe acting-out behavior. Over a period of several years, he improved remarkably in treatment and worked through a good deal of his abandonment depression, but, as time came for him to work through his separation from the therapist, he decided to leave the country and thereby provide the illusion of independence in his behavior, while he retained the intrapsychic image of the therapist.

Ten years later he returned to therapy in an abandonment depression because of the break-up of a love affair. His functioning had been extremely good since he ceased treatment, but his object relations had continued to be problematic. He had formed a clinging relationship with a younger, probably inappropriate, woman. When he proposed that she live with him, she told him she was too young but added that she wanted to continue seeing him. He was offended at the frustration of his wish for exclusive possession, dropped her and went into an abandonment depression. He resumed treatment but continued to defend himself against the depression by distancing, detachment and sexual acting-out which did not yield to confrontation. After about six months of treatment twice a week, he found the same pseudo solution to his problem—he found another girl, moved in, and immediately began to feel better and decided to stop treatment.

Jane K.

The second patient, Jane, 18, presented a history of depression, obesity, profuse heterosexual acting-out, and great difficulty in being on her own. She did well in the testing and working-through phase of her treatment, but as she came to the separation phase her temptation to resolve it by acting out mounted; as her separation anxiety rose, she began seeing a man and formed a relationship with him which did not yield to interpretations. She stopped treatment and married. Several years later she returned because of severe conflict with her husband, who was extremely negative and hostile to her, and she got a divorce. Over the next several years, up to age 28, her functioning continued intact at a high level, and she eventually established a professional life of her own. Her object relations continued at a level of great conflict. She had one after another abortive relationship with men, who always turned out to be inappropriate. After all this time, she finally returned to treatment to work on her problem in object relations. The biggest threat, the strongest precipitator of separation anxiety, was the possibility of a real, intimate relationship. She defended against this by assiduously avoiding appropriate men, ending up with transient affairs and then blaming the men for it.

Peter L.

Another example is Peter L., who, in the last stage of his treatment, not only had improved functionally and symptomatically, but also showed clear evidence of whole object relations in the transference, a consolidated feeling of self, and freedom of self-assertion, all of which were reflected in his life structure. However, it seemed clear that his urge to stop therapy was to avoid working through feelings of anxiety and depression about separation from his intrapsychic image of the therapist, that he wished to act out in order to retain this image and not have to face these feelings. Again, no amount of confrontation seemed to be effective, and since Peter showed the best functioning and feeling levels of his life, the therapist had no alternative but to go along with his wish to stop. In several phone calls approximately four years later, it appeared that his adaptation has continued at this high level.

Joan M.

The next patient, Joan M., 30, an executive, came for treatment in an abandonment panic when her husband declared that he wanted a divorce. She had a long history of conflictual relationships with men, including three marriages and several affairs. She often picked out unsuitable men and ended up feeling rejected and abandoned in the relationship. When intensely involved with a man, she felt extremely vulnerable and dependent and tended to be jealous, suspicious and clinging, while other times, when not involved, she was completely detached, could carry on extensive relationships involving mainly role-playing without affect.

Her psychodynamic structure and background were similar to Catherine's in that, in order to deal with the feelings of abandonment in the relationship with her mother, she had transferred the symbiotic image of the mother to the father, who became a target for the symbiotic projection. She complied with his expectations, denying the destructive aspect of the father's behavior. This complicated, intrapsychic structure was then carried out through relationships with a variety of men.

In six years of analysis, four times a week, much of her abandonment depression was worked through; there was again dramatic improvement in her functional capacity in her work, her interests, her creativity, her relationships in general, the area of relationships with men always standing out as an exception. She claimed that there were no eligible men available. She conducted a series of sterile relationships, where the men were more involved than she; she carried out the illusion of a relationship without the emotional involvement. Confrontation of this as a resistance, probably to transference feelings, made very little headway. However, the patient's life improved so dramatically, as shown in her work, her creativity, her interests, her social relationships, her activities—she was extraordinarily able and competent in all these areas—that she began to make an argument first for cutting down and eventually for stopping treatment. I vigorously objected each time, saying that we would have to disagree, that I thought she was doing it in order not to face some of these feelings and that it was my guess that if she terminated she would continue to have difficulty in her relationships with men.

Despite my caution she persisted, and at the end of the sixth year stopped treatment. In one of our discussions, I made a hypothesis: If she was right and I was wrong, she would eventually find someone, and the relationship would go quite smoothly; if I was right and she was wrong, either she would find no relationship or, if she found a realistic one and became emotionally involved, the relationship would bring out of hiding all the feelings that she was running away from by stopping treatment—probably fears of engulfment or abandonment.

The prediction came true when the patient returned five months later, overwhelmed with anxiety in the setting of having fallen in love and starting to live with a man. She reported that she was alright when they were together but when they were not she felt extremely vulnerable; she was very sensitive to the smallest stimuli, which would produce a suspicion that he didn't care about her, fear that he was abandoning her, and possessive, jealous rages, with feelings of depression and despair.

These feelings were either acted out with the man, in which case they were very destructive to the relationship, or the patient controlled them, feeling intense anxiety, anger and depression;

when she went to sleep, she would have nightmares of being attacked by the father and/or the mother. She also had dreams of telling the mother to get out of her life. This real-life involvement had tapped the deepest level of the patient's object relations, i.e., her fears of abandonment and engulfment associated not only with the symbiotic image projected on the father but with the original symbiotic relationship with the mother as well. She returned to treatment to finally work through this fundamental and ultimate tie.

This case illustrates how difficult it is to separate father's influence from mother's influence and, therefore, in treatment to remove the pathological effects of the relationship with the father without also working on the relationship with the mother. It casts grave doubt upon Kohut's assertion (63) that one can work through the compensatory structures of the father without having to deal with the conflict with the mother to get an optimum clinical result.

TERMINATION BECAUSE OF TRANSFERENCE ADDICTION

Some patients receive so much gratification in fantasy from the treatment that it amounts to an addiction, and the therapist can work until doomsday before these patients will initiate the idea of stopping treatment. It is important to recognize this feature as an indication for the therapist to initiate termination.

Case Illustrations

Leslie

Leslie, discussed in earlier chapters, after eight years of analysis, four times a week, had changed from an almost psychotic-like state to close to normal, adaptive functioning with minimum symptomatology. She had worked through an enormous amount of earlier preoedipal conflicts with the mother and father. However, her mother and father had additionally scapegoated her in the phallic, oedipal period so that her oedipal condensations were deely embedded, intense and sadomasochistic. After her adaptation improved, she moved into this oedipal phase of treatment with a principal defense of transference acting-out. Several years of analysis of the sadomasochistic, oedipal conflict, particularly of her loss of the caretaking and oedipal father and her transference acting-out defenses against it with me in sessions, again set free a good deal of sexual feeling and sexual desire.

However, although she was adapting in every other respect, the patient was procrastinating about dating and about extending her new sexual feeling into reality and action. She had survived her childhood traumas by almost totally investing her emotions in her fantasy life and holding reality in abeyance; thus, the use of fantasy, particularly transference acting-out in fantasy, had become her principal mode of behavior. Although this mode had disappeared in most areas, it was not yielding to working-through as one might expect.

As the content became repetitive, without much change, and as the patient became aware of the degree to which her seeing me so often was a powerful stimulus to fantasy which she could not control, we agreed to cut down the frequency of her sessions to once a week in an effort to reduce the gratification involved in the fantasies and thereby help her gain control of her feelings.

The patient did show some improvement, but over a period of years, she became aware that: "There's nothing left to analyze, but I don't act on it. I'm shocked by my behavior. I do nothing; I'm acting like a child. My head is full of angry fantasies—a woman both sadistic and masochistic. On the one hand, the man is the sadist, and I am the victim; the next moment, I'm the sadist and the man is the victim. It's all to get revenge on my parents through you." When I emphasized the need to set limits to these fantasies and that this need would be supported by real relationships, the anger turned more intensely into the transference. "I'm mad at you. You want me to do it myself. I'm furious that I have to do it myself. I'm angry that my father particularly did not support my being a woman, and I have to do it myself. And I can feel that I don't want to do it. My urge is to screw up my sex life to get back at him through you. The more I feel sexual pleasure, the more separate I feel, the more spite I feel, the more I want to get back. This puts a lock on my genitals. I won't have an orgasm just to get back at you for not supporting my femininity."

She finally concluded: "I have to stop treatment for a while to see if I can stop fantasizing about you as a parent and force myself to give up the fantasy; I realize I have to do it myself. I have been seeing you since I was 18. I know that I'm acting out with you an angry, revenge fantasy because you will not do it for me. I coopt all progress into this fantasy.

I suggested that she seemed almost addicted to this fantasy of having it done for her, which was partially fueled by the illusions created by the fact that I was her doctor whose job it was to treat her. She reported that she felt that she could do it, that the only thing that was keeping her back was the anger that she had to do it herself: "The benefits of not incorporating progress in this fantasy outweighed the motivation of leaving in anger at your not taking care of me."

It seems to me that the risk for this patient is that she will find a man to be a caretaking father-figure through whom she will continue to act out these fantasies, rather than set limits to them in order to grow.

Lynn

The final case is Lynn, the teacher reported in great detail in a prior volume (83). When she remarried, her symptoms cleared up, as did her adaptation. She had an extraordinarily stable and contented relationship with a man. She had received a number of promotions at work and mentioned some, easily containable anxiety about engulfment or abandonment in the relationship with the man. When she was being seen once a week, the content of her interview was repetitive, without much change, consisting mostly of reports of the events in her new job, very little emotional conflict or content. Finally she began to complain about the time it took to come for sessions. I brought all these things to her attention as her way of conveying to me that perhaps she no longer needed the treatment. She agreed but said that if I didn't bring it to her attention, she would never stop coming. She then agreed to stop. I have not heard from her in about a year, which suggests that her improvement has been maintained.

The termination phase of treatment recapitulates, works through and challenges the efficacy of all the treatment that has gone before. Its complexities require careful consideration and management.

III. Reflections

13

Reflections

This book has attempted to demonstrate how a developmental perspective, specifically that derived from recognition of the clinical vicissitudes of the arrests of development occurring during the stages of separation-individuation, provides a close and appropriate fit between theory and clinical evidence in narcissistic and borderline disorders which in turn leads to a more appropriate and effective treatment.

It has emphasized that particular and specific attention must be paid in the case of every borderline patient to the following triad: Faulty separation-individuation leads to depression, which leads to defense. This developmental sequence, or track, reflects the essence of the developmental arrest, provides the therapist with the most reliable guide, and should be the axis around which other clinical observations are organized.

Separation-individuation, a broad and technical term, does not accurately convey how specifically and uniquely the borderline triad operates and can be identified as operating in each patient. The individuation which unfolds from within is manifested clinically by the patient's identifying and implementing in reality his own thoughts, feelings and wishes. It is the self-assertive activation of these unique thoughts, wishes and feelings that triggers the abandonment depression, which triggers the defense. Often the patient's greatest resistance is in recognizing that "he feels bad because he is trying to express what he wants and what he feels."

The therapist's task is through confrontation to bring to the patient's awareness the intrapsychic operation of this borderline triad which impels the patient to control the self-destructive, defensive behavior. This in turn rekindles the patient's own separation-individuation process which activates the abandonment depression and thus provides the therapist with the opportunity to help the patient work through the vicissitudes of this painful state.

There are three critical clinical turning points in psychoanalytical psychotherapy of the borderline patient, each of which has its own specific vulnerabilities. The first critical turning point is the change in the patient's perception of the functioning of his pathological ego from ego-syntonic to ego-alien. Should this not occur, the patient inevitably will stop treatment. The second, in the working-through phase, is the mastery of the talionic impulse which frees aggression to support growth. Failure at this point will result in the perpetuation of the defense against the abandonment depression. The final critical turning point in the last phase of treatment is the identification and working-through of the anxiety at separation from the introjected image of the therapist. Failure at this turning point will result in a less-than-optimum result.

The etiology and psychodynamics of the narcissistic disorder are far less clear. Theoretically, the developmental arrest of the narcissistic disorder may occur before that of the borderline. In any event, the narcissistic defensive object relations fused-unit with its fused grandiose-self, omnipotent-object representation effectively blocks the patient's individuation, and the psychoanalytic psychotherapy then also has three critical clinical turning points similar to the borderline: The first, in the testing phase, is the patient's gradual awareness of the defensive function of his object relations fused-unit.

The vulnerability in this first stage is that the patient will react to the therapist's interventions as attacks and mobilize his defensive operations, denial and devaluation, which will prevent the developing of a therapeutic alliance and bring the psychotherapy to a halt. The second, in the working-through phase, is the painful working-through of the aggressive object relations fused-unit and its abandonment depression and fragmented self. Failure at this point also results in the perpetuation of the narcissistic defenses. The third turning point in the final or separation phase is the working through of the anxiety at separation from the therapist and achieving a full, autonomous self-representation.

The therapist's task is through interpretation of the patient's vulnerability to narcissistic wounds in the therapeutic relationship to bring to the patient's awareness the defensive function of his grandiose-self, omnipotent-object representations and the abandonment depression and fragmented self that lay beneath it. This leads him to working through the depression which in turn frees his true self to emerge.

PROBLEMS IN TREATMENT OF THE BORDERLINE AND NARCISSISTIC DISORDERS

Standard errors implementing these tasks can be found at opposite ends of the therapeutic spectrum: psychoanalytic psychotherapy and other more directive forms of therapy.

Psychoanalytic Psychotherapy

The first type of error is shown by many analysts (44-50) who use object relations theory in their work and who do perceive the borderline problem as being preoedipal. However, when they do not link their observations and interventions to the borderline triad—separation-individuation leads to depression which leads to defense—their treatment lacks a refined focus, as it is not anchored on the main axis of the patient's problem. For example, they might deal adequately with the patient's defenses and correctly identify and bring to the patient's attention his rage and depression, with their associated self- and object representations. But when they do not link these observations to the patient's individuation process, the treatment is left to wander and cannot develop the cohesive, integrating power that accurate interventions produce. You cannot say it is entirely wrong but that it falls too short of the mark.

The second type of error is shown by those analysts who seek to find their answers to these problems in classical instinctual theory and oedipal conflict, overlooking the earlier separation-individuation failure and ascribing the clinical consequences, the patient's depression, to oedipal conflict. They don't perceive how transference acting-out differs from transference, i.e., transference requires whole object relations, a stage these patients have not achieved. These therapists, therefore, are unable to apply the appropriate therapeutic interventions. They interpret rather than confront; the interpretations fall on deaf and unprepared ears, and treatment is ineffective.

Clear examples of this type of misperceptions of the borderline are seen in the review that follows of two analytic cases (17):

Shirley T.

The analyst's view that Shirley's problems were oedipal, that she had a strong masochistic character, was no doubt stimulated by Shirley's defense, consisting of sexual acting-out. The latter impelled the analyst to overestimate the oedipal features in her history and in the treatment to overlook the earlier and more fundamental borderline problem.

Thus, in eliciting her history, the analyst concentrated on sexual and other libidinal issues at phallic and oedipal levels. He mentions little or nothing about Shirley's relationship with her mother or the early development of the self, except to say that the mother was critical, bigoted and preferred the brother; he reports only incidentally and much later that Shirley had had allergic attacks in childhood and nocturnal anxiety attacks at age 13, which required the mother to share the bed with her. The history is not only incomplete but also seems to be distorted to fit the analyst's theoretical assumptions.

These misperceptions produced confusion in the treatment. The therapist's misconceiving of the transference as being based on the father rather than the mother endlessly confused his and later the husband's role in the patient's life and led him to interpret rather than confront. As a result, the treatment lacked sufficient depth.

In my view, appropriate treatment for Shirley required an understanding of the intrapsychic split object relations part-units of the borderline, the rewarding part-unit and the withdrawing part-unit, and how the patient defended against the latter by splitting, projection, and acting-out. Shirley was fixated in a symbiotic relationship with her mother. This fixation resulted in the two object relations part-units which were kept apart by the splitting defense. The rewarding object relations part-unit from the mother was then projected on the father, who became a symbol for the rewarding part-unit relationship with the mother rather than a father in his own right; i.e., the intrapsychic structure remained dyadic, not triadic. The withdrawing part-unit was projected back on the mother.

This defense was additionally complicated later on in the phallic and oedipal period by the guilt feelings aroused by the father's seductive behavior. The splitting, projection, and acting-out of the rewarding part-unit on men and the withdrawing part-unit back on mother or other men, in particular the analyst, became a way of life for Shirley.

She began analysis while having an affair. The rewarding part-unit continued to be projected upon the man with whom she was having the affair, while she acted out in the transference the withdrawing part-unit projections by attacking the analyst, thus repeating in analysis the splitting projection and acting-out defenses which began in her early relationship with her mother.

I think her anxiety that analysis might lead her to become psychotic expressed the feeling that, if she gave up the defense of splitting and acting-out of the withdrawing part-unit and contained it, she would feel engulfed by hostility and depression and become psychotic.

Further evidence of the alternate projection of the maternal rewarding and withdrawing object representation projections on the analyst was seen in the patient's intense separation anxiety when the therapist was away, leading her to have affairs with several men.

After about 18 months of treatment, she married, I suspect to institutionalize the splitting defense—in other words, to have one man there permanently in order to play him off against the other man, the analyst. She constantly titrated her involvement with her husband against her involvement with the analyst, who did not perceive that her handling of these two relationships represented opposite sides of the same coin. The only way she could relate to the analyst was a part-object (the RORU) which required another relationship on which to project her split WORU.

The confusion about this crucial split was illustrated by the analyst's interpreting that her hostility to him or the husband was a displacement from one to the other. Actually, both of these attitudes were pathological and both represented not displacements from one to the other but rather alternate projections of the same withdrawing object relations part-unit from the relationship with the mother. Therefore, it was necessary to confront the reality that both were inappropriate projections, thus impelling the patient to contain them in her psyche and attempt to work them through in treatment rather than act them out.

Shirley's transference acting-out derived from her projection of the rewarding part-unit on the father. The analyst then became a symbol for that father and the husband a symbol for the withdrawing object relations unit negative projections of the mother.

During her final sessions of treatment, the patient likened the grief she felt to that of giving up an affair with an ineligible man. There was much truth to this statement. Since her treatment had never touched upon the earlier relationship with the mother, had never worked through the abandonment depression, the ending of the analytic relationship was quite similar to the ending of one of her defensive affairs.

This confusion is further illustrated by Shirley's statement that she regarded her analyst as a protector against her husband. This seems to me to be a projection. The truth of the matter is the reverse; the husband was a protection against the analyst, serving as a target for the withdrawing part-unit projections. She could not decide on ending her marriage while the analysis was in progress. She probably could not decide because she still needed the husband as a defense against further involvement with the analyst. The question of separation from the husband also arose at the time of separation from the analyst; if she stopped seeing the analyst, she would no longer need the husband as a defense. Her yearnings for her analyst vacillated with the yearnings for her husband, both being defenses against overcoming her splitting defense and dealing with her hostile, withdrawing part-unit projections and working through her abandonment depression. For a clear illustration of how to deal with this kind of transference acting out, the reader can consult the management of Catherine in Chapter 12. She was confronted with her withdrawing and rewarding part-unit projections rather than having them interpreted as displacements.

Charlotte E.

The therapist viewed the patient's principal problem as being separation but did not utilize this insight for treatment of her transference acting-out. Charlotte displayed intense transference acting-out of the withdrawing object relations part-unit. At one point the therapist almost seemed to see the acting-out for what it was, except that he called it maternal transference rather than transference acting-out; at other times, he seemed to see it as a defense against oedipal conflict.

Charlotte was transference acting out the WORU to avoid a real relationship and involvement with the analyst, which would have produced containment of these angry feelings and a severe depression. The analyst, rather than use confrontation to convert the acting-out to working-through (introspection), tried only to "encourage" the patient to be introspective. When the patient is acting out, no amount of encouragement is going to produce introspection since the purpose of acting out is to avoid introspection. It is only through confrontation, with control of acting-out, that introspection emerges. When the therapist's "encouragements" failed, he proposed termination with the apparent aim of helping the patient come to grips with the projection and acting-out of aggression on the analyst.

The decision to terminate, i.e., to avoid involvement, by both analyst and patient, set limits to the struggle over involvement and thereby reduced the patient's anxiety; the withdrawing part-unit projection decreased, and to all appearances, the therapeutic alliance improved. Now that the patient was not going to have to get involved on the symbiotic level and deal with her negative projections, the analyst and she could "talk better" about her problems. In my view, effective therapy had ceased. Without confrontation, it took Charlotte five and one-half years to appreciate how rude she had been all the while to her analyst. A contrast, showing what I mean by the use of confrontation to deal with the withdrawing-unit projections, can be seen in the case of Fred (Chapters 7, 8, 9).

Gedo (34), commenting on these cases, made the following point: "The interpretation of the oedipus complex did not resolve the conflict, because the developmental antecedents had not been dealt with."

A similar example of the damage that ensues from misperceiving a narcissistic disorder as being related to oedipal conflict is seen in the following report of a patient seen in consultation.

John A.

A 48-year-old, successful, divorced professional man came for consultation to evaluate the progress of his eight years of analysis, four times a week. Quite typically, he did not come of his own volition, because he was dissatisfied, but at the urging of his latest girlfriend and her therapist, whom he had also been seeing in couples therapy. He had divorced two wives because "they weren't perfect enough," and when trouble developed with his current girlfriend, she suggested they see her therapist together. Her therapist, astonished at the small amount of improvement the patient reported from his analysis, suggested a consultation.

He had started analysis because of 1) his overwhelming need to be perfect, 2) his search for a perfect woman, which always seemed to meet failure, 3) the rigidity of his conscience and the lack of awareness of his feeling states, 4) his inability to accept any criticism to which he reacted with rage and withdrawal, 5) his intolerance of the shortcomings of others, 6) his unending need for approval, 7) sexual difficulties leading to impotence when in conflict with a woman. After eight years, all the above were still present but, in his view, somewhat reduced in intensity. He lauded the excellence (perfection) of his analyst and knew him to be (as he indeed was) at the top of the profession. He was very impressed by the "brilliance" of his analyst's interpretations of his dreams. However, at the same time, the patient also recognized in himself that he consciously avoided bringing up conflictual material with the analyst, was often late for interviews or missed them with flimsy excuses and none of this bothered him. Beyond that, his analyst never confronted these issues.

Further questioning revealed that his view of his parents was little changed from that of childhood. His mother was "vain, beautiful, loving," and his father "successful and perfect." When I investigated further the course of the analysis, he reported that he had never experienced substantial periods of depression and had never felt attacked by or in conflict with his analyst as he had with practically everyone else, and this didn't bother him either.

It seems to me that this is a good example of a narcissistic therapist and a narcissistic patient "sharing" their narcissistic glow at the cost of progress in treatment.

How are we to explain the perpetuation of these errors by otherwise able therapists? Freud staked out the boundaries of normal preoedipal development and the possible psychopathology that could stem from this early period. He then moved on to concentrate his life's work on the consequences of oedipal conflict for the development of neuroses. Some of his followers, less independent and less flexible, developed a dogmatic insistence upon oedipal conflict as being not only the primary source of emotional conflict, which of course it is, but the sole source, with other possible preoedipal determinants being almost completely devalued.

The work of those who undertook to study preoedipal sources of difficulty, such as Melanie Klein (54-57) with children and Guntrip (37) and Fairbairn (15) with adults, was similarly devalued and isolated from the mainstream. This led to an artificial conflict between these two points of view which, although somewhat lessened, persists vigorously to this day, much to the detriment of patients with developmental arrests.

The work in this volume on the psychopathology that springs from the separation-individuation failure obviously falls within the preoedipal area and consequently comes under the same kinds of attack from this source. Those who feel that their global and exclusive notions about the importance of the oedipal conflict are being threatened devalue notions with regard to separation-individuation and continue to overlook these factors in their borderline and narcissistic patients. As a result, the treatment suffers.

This argument, it seems to me, rather unwisely and arbitrarily stresses that either oedipal or preoedipal factors are the sole contributors to emotional conflicts. It seems to me that they both make their own contribution, the major preoedipal contribution being to the borderline and narcissistic disorders or developmental arrests, the main oedipal contribution being to the neuroses. This does not mean that the preoedipal factors do not contribute to the neuroses or that the oedipal factor does not contribute to the developmental arrest; it is a matter of degree.

These same people, while ignoring the preoedipal evidence to fit the patient into their oedipal theories, under the guise of "remaining neutral" or "avoiding closure," as so often happens, turn around and accuse those of us who emphasize preoedipal factors of doing the same thing—fitting the patient into the procrustean bed of our own theories and overlooking other important aspects of the problem, particularly oedipal conflict. Obviously, all therapists have to be constantly on guard against their own tendencies to bias and prejudice, as it happens from time to time to the best. And they must constantly check and recheck their clinical hypotheses. However, within this caution, it seems to me that this view is based on a failure to appreciate the specificity of both the borderline triad and the defensive fused-unit of the narcissistic disorder. Most treatment failures that I have seen have been not from an overlooking of other aspects of the patient's problem, but from a failure to perceive and concentrate adequately on these crucial features.

The argument that oedipal conflict will be overlooked reflects a lack of understanding of the psychopathology of the developmental arrest. As demonstrated in the cases of Ann and Leslie, as the patient works through the abandonment depression and growth resumes, the patient logically and in the expected developmental sequence moves from the separation-individuation failure into a condensed oedipal conflict. To try to deal with the latter before resolving the former would put the cart before the horse.

More Directive Therapies

Some therapists of this persuasion provide an excess of external structure, i.e., directions, advice, etc., for patients, which sometimes allows them to organize their lives better and to feel affects that many have never felt before; however, the presence of the external structure, so useful for enabling the patient to function better, at the same time prevents the patient from individuating. The rewarding object relations part-unit of the borderline and the defensive fused-unit of the narcissistic disorder become activated, and progress in treatment stops. One cannot direct or force a patient to individuate. The more one attempts to take over this responsibility for the patient, the more one prevents individuation. Individuation proceeds from within. The therapist with a borderline or narcissistic patient, as a servant of this process, can only create the conditions which make separation-individuation possible. If it is to emerge, the patient has to and will take it from there on his own.

Some Other Objections

Kernberg objected to my view of the borderline as being an oversimplification (48), perhaps because he does not perceive the clinical specificity of the borderline triad. He also misinterprets my concept of confrontive or supportive psychotherapy as requiring guidance and direction and, therefore, causing the therapist to abandon his stance of therapeutic neutrality. The difference between confrontive and intensive analytic psychotherapy is mainly one of objectives. Confrontive psychoanalytic psychotherapy does not try to work through the abandonment depression, while analytic psychotherapy does. In confrontive therapy, the therapist maintains his objective stance but relies more on confrontation than interpretation.

Gunderson (39), engaged in the necessary but laborious task of establishing research methodology to answer some of these clinical questions, raised the question as to whether what I have called "the abandonment depression" actually exists. Since the full impact of the abandonment depression only reveals itself in the working-through phase of psychoanalytic psychotherapy as the defenses are worked through, it is not surprising that the author, who deals mainly with modern research methodology and not with working-through defenses, continues to have his doubts. Unless he had worked through the borderline patient's defenses properly, the abandonment depression would not emerge fully, and he would continue to question its existence, while it flourished hidden behind the patient's defenses.

THE PURPOSE OF PSYCHOTHERAPY

The purpose of the treatment is not insight—to make the unconscious conscious—but rather to promote the reliving of old experiences by the more mature psyche, to discharge and work through the abandonment depression, which resulted from parental failures to support growth, thereby freeing the self-representation to separate from the object representation.

Psychotherapy, through its requirement that the patient assume responsibility for the initiation, identification and reporting of his feeling states—in other words, he must assume responsibility for the emotional state of the self and its expression, or if not, examine why not—rekindles the separation-individuation process and immediately brings the patient in the interview up against all the difficulties which have created this defect in the structure of the self in the first place—his need to defend against the abandonment depression that separation-individuation induces. The psychotherapy becomes itself an experiment in individuation. In the therapeutic crucible, when the patient activates his usual defenses, such as avoidance or transference acting-out, these are dealt with by the therapist by confrontation and/or other techniques which refocus and provide a framework for the patient to work through his abandonment depression or reexperience the disappointment, anger and depression that helped to produce the defect in the first place.

As these affects are discharged, other features of the psychotherapy support the patient's further growth:

1) the consistent regular reliability of the therapist;
2) the dyadic character of the relationship, which reinforces the patient's symbiotic projections but also intensifies the

patient's availability to introjection once projections have been dealt with;

3) the therapist's activities:

(a) *listening, understanding*—potent forces which the patient initially sees as a threat, since these experiences of human empathy are often the first the patient has been aware of. They bring with them, by dramatic contrast, the extraordinary pain of the early parental failures in empathy;

(b) *confrontation*—which does for the patient what he is unable to do for himself because of ego defects and pathologic defense mechanisms (avoidance, denial, projection, projective identification), i.e., perceive reality. The patient identifies with the therapist and then learns to perform this function for himself;

(c) *interpretation*—which broadens understanding and enhances control;

(d) *communicative matching*—which provides the responsive, sharing experience with the patient's new individuative thoughts, feelings and actions, compensating for the defect left by mother's withdrawal and fuels and invigorates the patient's individuation.

These therapeutic activities over time establish a harmonious emotional rhythm which meets the patient's emotional therapeutic needs in a manner resembling the optimal mother-child emotional interaction during the crucial symbiotic separation-individuation phases of development. They are not the same—one meets therapeutic needs, the other basic emotional needs for love, support, etc.—but the former resembles the latter in its regularity, consistency, availability of the therapist and the constructive effect of his actions.

This state of affairs potentiates the patient's working-through of his abandonment depression, as well as his use of the therapist as an object for positive introjections, all of which facilitate individuation and the overcoming of the developmental arrest.

These results go far toward laying to rest, it seems to me, the notion that borderline and narcissistic patients cannot benefit from developmentally based psychoanalytic psychotherapy. The therapy is arduous, time-consuming, filled with seductive and deceptive obstacles, but it is far from impossible. When it is pursued faithfully, it more than justifies the effort, providing, as it does, a life preserver to rescue and sustain the deprived and abandoned in their struggle and eventually a beacon to guide them to overcome their developmental trauma, reconstruct their psyche, and rejoin the mainstreams of life. These objectives—a fulfillment of both the therapist's and patient's deepest wishes—enhance the mutual struggle and endow it with a vitality and nobility that gives the work its enduring satisfaction and significance.

Bibliography

1. ABELIN, E. "The Role of the Father in the Separation-Individuation Process," in: Settlage, C. F. and McDevitt, J. B. (Eds.), *Separation-Individuation—Essays in Honor of Margaret S. Mahler.* New York: Int. Univ. Press, 229-251, 1971.
2. ABELIN, E. "Triangulation, The Role of the Father and the Origins of Core Gender Identity During the Rapprochement Subphase," in: *Rapprochement—The Central Subphase of Separation-Individuation.* New York: Jason Aronson, Inc., 1980.
2a. AMERICAN PSYCHIATRIC ASSOCIATION. *Diagnostic and Statistical Manual (Third Edition).* Washington, D.C., 1980.
3. BENEDEK, T. "Adaptation of Reality in Early Infancy," *Psa. Quart.,* 7:200-215, 1938.
4. BENEDEK, T. "Parenthood As A Developmental Phase," *J. Amer. Psa. Assn.,* 7:389-417, 1959.
5. BENEDEK, T. "The Psychosomatic Implications of the Primary Unit: Mother-Child," *Amer. J. Orthopsychiat.,* 19:642-654, 1949.
6. BENEDEK, T. "Psychobiological Aspects of Mothering," *Amer. J. Orthopsychiat.,* 26:272-278, 1956.
7. BOWLBY, J. *Attachment and Loss, Vol. I, Attachment.* New York: Basic Books, 1969.

235

8. BOWLBY, J. *Attachment and Loss, Vol. II, Separation.* New York: Basic Books, 1973.
9. BOWLBY, J. "Grief and Mourning in Infancy and Early Childhood," *Psa. Study Child,* 15:9-52, 1960.
10. BOWLBY, J. "Process of Mourning," *Int. J. Psa.,* 42:317-340, 1961.
11. BOWLBY, J. "Separation Anxiety." *Int. J. Psa.,* 41:89-113, 1960.
12. BOWLBY, J. "The Nature of the Child's Tie to His Mother," *Int. J. Psa.,* 39: 350-371, 1958.
13. EISNITZ, A. "On the Metapsychology of Narcissistic Pathology," *J. Amer. Psa. Assn.,* Vol. 22:2, 1974.
14. EISNITZ, A. "Narcissistic Object Choice and Self-Representation," *Int. J. Psa.,* 50:15-25, 1969. Discussed in *Int. J. Psa.,* 51:151-157, 1970.
15. FAIRBAIRN, W. R. "A Revised Psychopathology of the Psychoses and Psychoneuroses," in: *Psychoanalytic Studies of the Personality (An Object Relations Theory of the Personality).* London: Tavistock, 1952; New York: Basic Books, 1954.
16. FEDERN, P. *Ego Psychology and the Psychoses.* New York: Basic Books, 1952.
17. FIRESTEIN, S. *Termination in Psychoanalysis.* New York: Int. Univ. Press, 1978.
18. FRAIBERG, S. "Libidinal Object Constancy and Mental Representation," *Psa. Study Child,* 24:9-47, 1969.
19. FREIDMAN, H. "Current Psychoanalytic Object Relations Theory and Its Clinical Implications," *Int. J. Psa.,* 56:137-146, 1975.
20. FREUD, S. "Civilization and Its Discontents," *The Standard Edition of the Complete Psychological Works of S. Freud.* London: The Hogarth Press, Vol. XXI; pp. 64-109, 1955.
21. FREUD, S. "Fetishism" (1927), in: Strachey, J. (Ed.), *Collected Papers, Vol. V.* London: Hogarth Press, 198-204, 1950.
22. FREUD, S. "Further Recommendations in the Technique of Psychoanalysis: Recollection, Repetition and Working Through." *Collected Papers, Vol. II.* London: Hogarth Press, 1953. pp. 366-376.
23. FREUD, S. "Formulations on the Two Principles of Mental Functioning," in: *Standard Edition,* 12:218-226, 1911.
24. FREUD, S. "Instincts and Their Vicissitudes," (1915), *Standard Edition,* 14:117-140. London: The Hogarth Press, 1967.
25. FREUD, S. "On Narcissism: An Introduction," (1914), *Standard Edition,* 14:73-102. London: Hogarth Press, 1957.
26. FREUD, S. "Splitting of the Ego in the Defensive Process" (1938) in: Strachey, J. (Ed.), *Collected Papers, Vol. V.* London: Hogarth Press, 372-375, 1950.
27. FREUD, S. "Totems and Taboo," *The Standard Edition of the Complete Psychological Works of S. Freud.* London: Hogarth Press, Vol. XIII; pp. 1-100, 1955.
28. FREUD, A. and DANN, S. "An Experiment in Group Upbringing," *Psa. Study Child,* 6:127-168, 1951.
29. FROSCH, J. "Psychoanalytic Considerations of the Psychotic Character," *J. Amer. Psa. Assn.,* 15:606-625, 1967.
30. FROSCH, J. "Severe Regressive States During Analysis Summary," *J. Amer. Psa. Assn.,* 15:606-625, 1967.
31. FROSCH, J. "The Psychotic Character: Clinical Psychiatric Consideration," *J. Psych. Quart.,* 38:81-96, 1964.
32. FRYLING-SCHREUDER, E. C. "Borderline States in Children," *Psa. Study Child,* 11:336-351, 1956.

33. GABRIEL, E. "Analytic Group Psychotherapy With Borderline Psychotic Women," *Int. J. Group Psychother.*, 1:243-253, 1951.
34. GEDO, J. "Reflections on Some Current Controversies in Psychoanalysis," *J. Amer. Psa. Assn.*, Vol. 28, 1980. #2.
35. GIOVACCHINI, P. *Treatment of Primitive Mental States*. New York: Jason Aronson, Inc., 1979.
36. GOLDFARB, W. "Psychological Privation in Infancy and Subsequent Adjustment," *Amer. J. Orthopsychiat.*, 15:247-255, 1945.
36a. GROTSTEIN, J. *Splitting and Projective Identification*. New York: Aronson, 1981.
37. GUNTRIP, H. *Personality Structure and Human Interaction*. London: Hogarth Press; New York: Int. Univ. Press, 1964.
38. GUNTRIP, H. *Schizoid Phenomena, Object Relations and the Self*. New York: Int. Univ. Press, 1968.
39. GUNDERSON, J. G. and SINGER, M. T. "Defining Borderline Patients: An Overview," *Amer. J. Psych.*, 132:1-9, 1975.
40. JACOBSON, E. "Denial and Repression," *J. Amer. Psa. Assn.*, 5:61-92, 1957.
41. JACOBSON, E. *The Self and the Object World*. New York: Int. Univ. Press, 1964.
42. KAPLAN, L. *Rapprochement and Oedipal Organization: Effects on Borderline Phenomena in Rapprochement*. New York: Jason Aronson, Inc., 1980.
43. KERNBERG, O. "A Psychoanalytic Classification of Character Pathology, *J. Amer. Psa. Assn.*, 18:800-822, 1970.
44. KERNBERG, O. *Borderline Conditions and Pathological Narcissism*. New York: Science House, 163-177, 1975.
45. KERNBERG, O. "Borderline Personality Organization," *J. Amer. Psa. Assn.*, 15: 641-685, 1967.
46. KERNBERG, O. "Contrasting Approaches to the Psychotherapy of Borderline Conditions," in: James Masterson (Ed.), *New Perspectives on Psychotherapy of the Borderline Adult*. New York: Brunner/Mazel, 1978.
47. KERNBERG, O. "Contrasting Viewpoints Regarding the Nature and Psychoanalytic Treatment of Narcissistic Personalities: A Preliminary Communication," *Amer. J. Psa. Assn.*, 22:255-267, 1974.
48. KERNBERG, O. "Developmental Theory, Structural Organization and Psychoanalytic Technique," in *Rapprochement*. New York: Jason Aronson, Inc., 1980.
49. KERNBERG, O. "Further Considerations of the Treatment of Narcissistic Personalities," *Int. J. Psa.*, 55:215-240, 1974.
50. KERNBERG, O. "The Treatment of Patients With Borderline Personality Organization," *Int. J. Psa.*, 49:600-619, 1968.
51. KHAN, M. M. "Dread of Surrender to Resourceless Dependence in the Analytic Situation," in: *The Privacy of the Self*. New York: Int. Univ. Press, 270-279, 1974.
52. KHAN, M. M. "The Finding and Becoming of Self," in: *The Privacy of the Self*. New York: Int. Univ. Press, 294-305, 1974.
53. KLEIN, D. "Psychopharmacological Treatment and Delineation of Borderline Disorders" in: *Borderline Personality Disorders: The Concept, The Syndrome, The Patient*, P. Hartocallis (Ed.). New York: 1977.
54. KLEIN, M. "Contribution to the Psychogenesis of Manic Depressive States," in: *Contributions to Psychoanalysis* (1921-1945). London: Hogarth Press, 1948.
55. KLEIN, M. "Mourning and Its Relation to Manic Depressive States," in: *Contributions to Psychoanalysis* (1921-1945). London: Hogarth Press, 1948.

56. KLEIN, M. "Notes on Some Schizoid Mechanisms," in: Riviere, J. (Ed.), *Developments in Psychoanalysis*. London: Hogarth Press, 1946.
57. KLEIN, M. *The Psychoanalysis of Children*. London: Hogarth Press, 1932.
58. KOHUT, H. "Autonomy and Integration," *J. Amer. Psa. Assn.*, 13:851-856, 1965.
59. KOHUT, H. "Forms and Transformations of Narcissism," *J. Amer. Psa. Assn.*, 14:243-272, 1966.
60. KOHUT, H. "Panel on Narcissistic Resistance," (N. Segal, Reporter), *J. Amer. Psa. Assn.*, 17:941-954, 1969.
61. KOHUT, H. "Psychoanalytic Treatment of Narcissistic Personality Disorder: Outline of A Systematic Approach," *Psa. Study Child*, 23:86-113, 1968.
62. KOHUT, H. *The Analysis of the Self: A Systematic Approach to the Psychoanalytic Treatment of Narcissistic Personality Disorders*. New York: Int. Univ. Press, 1971.
63. KOHUT, H. *The Restoration of the Self*. New York: Int. Univ. Press, 1977.
64. LICHTENSTEIN, H. "Identity and Sexuality: A Study of Their Interrelationship in Man," *J. Amer. Psa. Assn.*, 9:179-260, 1961.
65. LIDZ, T. *The Origin and Treatment of Schizophrenic Disorders*. New York: Basic Books, 1973.
66. LITTLE, M. "Countertransference and the Patient's Response to It," *Int. J. Psa.*, 32:32-40, 1951.
67. LITTLE, M. "On Basic Unity," *Int. J. Psa.*, 41:377-384, 1960.
68. LITTLE, M. "On Delusional Transference," *Int. J. Psa.*, 39:134-138, 1958.
69. LITTLE, M. "Transference in Borderline States," *Int. J. Psa.*, 47:476-485, 1966.
70. MACK, J. (Ed.). *Borderline States*. New York: Grune & Stratton, 1975.
71. MAENCHEN, A. "Object Cathexis in A Borderline Twin," *Psa. Study Child*, 23:438-456, 1968.
72. MAHLER, M. "A Study of the Separation-Individuation Process and Its Possible Application to Borderline Phenomena in the Psychoanalytic Situation," *Psa. Study Child*, 26:403-424, 1971.
73. MAHLER, M. "Autism and Symbiosis—Two Extreme Disturbances of Identity," *Int. J. Psa.*, 39:77-83, 1958.
74. MAHLER, M. *On Human Symbiosis and the Vicissitudes of Individuation*. New York: Int. Univ. Press, 1968.
75. MAHLER, M. "On the Significance of the Normal Separation-Individuation Phase," in: Schur, M. (Ed.), *Drives, Affects and Behavior, Vol. 2*. New York: Int. Univ. Press, 161-169, 1965.
76. MAHLER, M. *The Psychological Birth of the Human Infant*. New York: Basic Books, 1975.
77. MAHLER, M. "Thoughts About Development and Individuation," *Psa. Study Child*, 18:307-324, 1963.
78. MAHLER, M. and FURER, M. "Certain Aspects of the Separation-Individuation Phase," *Psa. Quart.*, 32:1-14, 1963.
79. MAHLER, M. and KAPLAN, L. "Developmental Aspects in the Assessment of Narcissistic and So-Called Borderline Personalities," in: *Borderline Personality Disorders: The Concept, The Syndrome, The Patient*, edited by P. Hartocallis. New York: Int. Univ. Press, 1977.
80. MAHLER, M. and LAPERRIERE, R. "Mother-Child Interactions During Separation-Individuation," *Psa. Quart.*, 34:483-489, 1965.
81. MAHLER, M. and McDEVITT, J. "Observations on Adaptation and Defense in Statu Nascendi," *Psa. Quart.*, 37:1-21, 1968.
82. MAHLER, M., PINE, F. and BERGMAN, A. "The Mother's Reaction to Her

Toddler's Drive For Individuation," in: Anthony, E. and Benedek, T. (Eds.), *Parenthood*. Boston: Little, Brown, 1970.

83. MASTERSON, J. *Psychotherapy of the Borderline Adult: A Developmental Approach*. New York: Brunner/Mazel, 1976.

84. MASTERSON, J. "The Splitting Defense Mechanism of the Borderline Adolescent: Developmental and Clinical Aspects," in: Mack, J. (Ed.), *Borderline States*. New York: Grune & Stratton, 1975.

85. MASTERSON, J. "Therapeutic Alliance and Transference," *Amer. J. Psychiatry*, 135:4, 437-441, 1978.

86. MASTERSON, J. *Treatment of the Borderline Adolescent: A Developmental Approach*. New York: John Wiley & Sons, Inc. 1972.

87. MASTERSON, J. with COSTELLO, J. *From Borderline Adolescent to Functioning Adult: The Test of Time*. New York: Brunner/Mazel, 1980.

88. MASTERSON, J. and RINSLEY, D. "The Borderline Syndrome: The Role of the Mother in the Genesis and Psychic Structure of the Borderline Personality," *Int. J. Psa.*, 56:163-178, 1975.

89. McDEVITT, J. "Separation-Individuation and Object Constancy," *J. Amer. Psa. Assn.*, 23:713-742, 1975.

90. MEISSNER, W., S.J. *Differential Diagnosis of Narcissistic Personalities From Borderline Conditions*, presented Amer. Psa. Assn., May, 1979, Chicago.

91. NIETZSCHE, F. *The Birth of Tragedy and the Genealogy of Morals*. Translated by Francis Golffing. New York: Doubleday, Garden City, 1955.

92. PIAGET, J. *Play, Dream and Imitation in Childhood*. New York: Norton, 1951.

93. PIAGET, J. *The Construction of Reality in the Child*. New York: Basic Books, 1954.

94. PIAGET, J. *The Psychology of Intelligence*. London: Routledge and Kegan, P., 1950.

95. PINE, F. "On the Expansion of the Affect Array: A Developmental Description," in: R. Lax, S. Back, J. Burland (Eds.), *Rapprochement*. New York: Jason Aronson, Inc., 1980.

96. RINSLEY, D. "An Object Relations View of Borderline Personality," presented at "The Internat'l Meeting on Borderline Disorders," The Menninger Foundation & The Nat'l Institute of Mental Health, Topeka, Kansas, 1976.

97. RINSLEY, D. "Economic Aspects of the Object Relations," *Int. J. Psa.*, 49:38-48, 1968.

98. RINSLEY, D. "Residential Treatment of Adolescents," in: Arieti, S. (Ed.), *American Handbook of Psychiatry, Second Revised Ed., Vol. II*. New York: Basic Books, 353-366, 1974.

99. RINSLEY, D. and CARTER, L. "Vicissitudes of Empathy in A Borderline Adolescent." To be published, *Int. J. Psa.*

99a. ROBINS, L. *Deviant Children Grown Up*. Baltimore: Williams and Wilkins, 1966.

100. ROTHSTEIN, ARNOLD, "An Explanation of the Diagnosis of the Narcissistic Personality Disorder," *J. Amer. Psa. Assn.*, Vol. 27, #4, pp. 893-912, 1979.

101. SCHWARTZ, L. "Narcissistic Personality Disorders—A Clinical Discussion," *J. Amer. Psa. Assn.*, 22:292-306, New York: Int. Univ. Press, 1974.

102. SPITZ, R. "Anaclitic Depression," *Psa. Study Child*, 2:313-341, 1946.

103. SPITZ, R. "Hospitalism: An Inquiry Into the Genesis of Psychiatric Conditions of Early Childhood," *Psa. Study Child*, 1:53-74, 1945.

104. SPITZ, R. "Hospitalism: A Follow-Up Report," *Psa. Study Child*, 2:303-342, 1946.

105. Spitz, R. "Relevancy of Direct Infant Observations," *Psa. Study Child*, 5:66-75, 1950.
106. Spitz, R. "The Evolution of Dialogue," in: Schur, M. (Ed.), *Drives, Affects, Behavior, Second Ed.* New York: Int. Univ. Press, 170-190, 1965.
107. Spitz, R. *The First Year of Life (A Psychoanalytic Study of Normal and Deviant Development of Object Relations).* New York: Int. Univ. Press, 1965.
108. Spitz, R. "The Smiling Response: A Contribution to the Ontogenesis of Social Relations," *Genet. Psychol. Monog., Vol. 34.* Provincetown, Mass.: Journal Press, 1957.
109. Spitz, R. *No and Yes.* New York: Int. Univ. Press, 1957.
110. Spruiell, Vann. "Theories of the Treatment of Narcissistic Personalities," *J. Amer. Psa. Assn.*, 22:268-278, New York: Int. Univ. Press, 1974.
111. Stone, M. H. *The Borderline Syndrome: Constitution, Personality, and Adaptation.* New York: McGraw Hill, 1980.
112. *The Holy Bible, Confraternity Version.* New York: Benzinger Bros., 1961.
113. Tuchman, Barbara. *A Distant Mirror.* New York: A Knopf, Inc., 1978.
114. Wangh, M. "Concluding Remarks on Technique and Prognosis in the Treatment of Narcissism," *J. Amer. Psa. Assn.*, 22:307-309, New York: Int. Univ. Press, 1974.
115. Weil, A. *Maturational Variations and Genetic-Dynamic Issues. J. Amer. Psa. Assn., Vol. 26, 1978. #3*
116. Weil, A. "The Basic Core," *Psa. Study Child*, 25:442-460, 1970.
117. Winnicott, D. "Ego Distortions in Terms of True and False Self," in: *The Maturational Processes and the Facilitating Environment.* New York: Int. Univ. Press, 140-152, 1965.
118. Winnicott, D. "Ego Integration in Child Development," in: *The Maturational Processes and the Facilitating Environment.* New York: Int. Univ. Press, 56-63, 1965.
119. Winnicott, D. "From Dependence Towards Independence in the Development of the Individual," in: *The Maturational Processes and the Facilitating Environment.* New York: Int. Univ. Press, 83-92, 1965.
120. Winnicott, D. "The Capacity to Be Alone," in: *The Maturational Processes and the Facilitating Environment.* New York: Int. Univ. Press, 29-36, 1965.
121. Winnicott, D. "The Development of the Capacity For Concern," in: *The Maturational Processes and the Facilitating Environment.* New York: Int. Univ. Press, 73-82, 1965.
122. Zetzel, E. R. "Anxiety and the Capacity to Bear It (1949)," in: *The Capacity For Emotional Growth.* New York: Int. Univ. Press, 33-52, 1970.
123. Zetzel, E. "Depressive Illness (1960), in: *The Capacity For Emotional Growth.* New York: Int. Univ. Press, 53-62, 1970.
124. Zetzel, E. "On the Incapacity to Bear Depression (1965)," in: *The Capacity For Emotional Growth.* New York: Int. Univ. Press, 82-114, 1970.
125. Zetzel, B. "The Analytic Situation and the Analytic Process," in: *The Capacity For Emotional Growth.* New York: Int. Univ. Press, pp. 197-215, 1970.
126. Zetzel, E. "The Concept of Transference (1956)," in: *The Capacity For Emotional Growth.* New York: Int. Univ. Press, 168-181, 1970.
127. Zetzel, E. "The Depressive Position (1953)," in: *The Capacity For Emotional Growth.* New York: Int. Univ. Press, 63-81, 1970.
128. Zetzel, E. "Therapeutic Alliance in the Analysis of Hysteria (1958)," in: *The Capacity For Emotional Growth.* New York: Int. Univ. Press, 182-196, 1970.

Index

Abandonment, 38, 150
  and depression, 13-17, 20, 24, 27, 41,
    42, 70, 76, 79, 80, 88-89, 103, 105,
    106, 107, 131, 133-37, 142, 144, 163,
    166, 169, 173, 179, 180, 187-88, 191,
    201, 205, 206, 209, 210, 220, 221, 225,
    229, 231, 232
  fears of, 46-48, 197, 198, 213, 215
Abreaction, 149
Acting-out, 42-48, 53, 54, 81, 106, 107, 110,
    111, 112, 116, 134, 136, 144, 199
  of adolescents, 42, 44
  and introspection, 226
  passive-aggressive, 190-91
  sexual, 11, 37, 123, 171, 206, 210, 222-23
  and termination of treatment, 197, 201,
    204-13
  and transference, xii, 30, 31, 32, 56, 57,
    59, 60, 62, 64, 67-68, 70, 73-74, 76,

    78-79, 83, 94, 97, 108, 133, 134, 135,
    148-52, 158, 160, 165-81, 214, 224,
    225, 231
Adaptation, 3, 7-8, 30, 44, 103, 104, 118-19,
    135, 176, 181, 192, 193, 197
Addiction to infantile gratification, 23
Adolescents, 135, 138, 195. *See also*
    Children
  acting-out of, 42, 44
  and borderline mothers, 132
  intensive therapy of, 209
  self in, 99
Affective disorder, 40, 42-43
Aggression, 16, 17-18, 27, 29, 220, 226. *See
    also* Rage
  and fused-units, 53-55, 59, 62, 68, 69,
    77, 79
  inhibition of, 142-43
  talionic, 185-89, 192

241

James F. Masterson, M.D., is Director of The Masterson Group for the Treatment of Character Disorders (Adult and Adolescent) and of The Character Disorder Foundation for Teaching and Research on the Character Disorders. In Addition, he is Clinical Professor of Psychiatry, Cornell University Medical College-New York Hospital (Payne Whitney Clinic).

This Volume advances theory and treatment originally set forth in Dr. Masterson's *Psychotherapy of the Borderline Adult.* He is also the author of over 60 journal articles and three widely acclaimed books: *The Psychiatric Dilemma of Adolescence, Treatment of the Borderline Adolescent: A Developmental Approach, and From Borderline Adolescent to Functioning Adult: The Test of Time.*